ADVANCES IN

Cardiac Surgery®

VOLUME 12

ADVANCES IN

Cardiac Surgery®

VOLUMES 1 THROUGH 9 (OUT OF PRINT)

VOLUME 10

VOLUME 11

ADVANCES IN

Cardiac Surgery®

VOLUME 12

Editor-in-Chief
Robert B. Karp, M.D.
Professor of Surgery, Chief of Cardiac Surgery, University of Chicago,
Pritzker School of Medicine, Chicago, Illinois

Editorial Board
Hillel Laks, M.D.
Professor and Chief, Division of Cardiothoracic Surgery; Director, Heart
and Heart–Lung Transplant Program, UCLA Medical Center, Los
Angeles, California

Andrew S. Wechsler, M.D.
Professor and Chairman, Department of Cardiothoracic Surgery,
Allegheny University of the Health Sciences, MCP Hahnemann School
of Medicine, Philadelphia, Pennsyivania

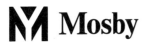 Mosby

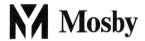

Publisher: Susan Patterson
Associate Publisher: Cynthia Baudendistel
Developmental Editor: Sarah A. Zagarri
Manager, Periodical Editing: Kirk Swearingen
Production Editor: Stephanie M. Geels
Project Supervisor, Production: Joy Moore
Composition Specialist: Laura Bayless

Printed in the United States of America
Printing/binding the by Maple-Vail Book Manufacturing Group

Editorial Office:
Mosby, Inc.
11830 Westline Industrial Drive
St. Louis, MO 63146

International Standard Serial Number: 0889-5074
International Standard Book Number: 0-8151-2726-X

Contributors

Juan C. Alejos, MD
Assistant Professor of Pediatrics, Division of Pediatric Cardiology, UCLA School of Medicine, Los Angeles, California

Anil Z. Apaydin, MD
Chief Resident in Cardiothoracic Surgery, Mount Sinai School of Medicine, New York, New York

Solomon Aronson, MD, FCCP
Associate Professor, Department of Anesthesia and Critical Care, University of Chicago; Director of Cardiothoracic Anesthesia, University of Chicago Hospitals, Chicago, Illinois

Caron Burch, RN, MSN
Division of Cardiothoracic Surgery, UCLA School of Medicine, Los Angeles, California

Ralph J. Damiano, Jr, MD
Professor and Chief, Department of Cardiothoracic Surgery, Pennsylvania State University; Chief, Section of Cardiothoracic Surgery, Penn State Geisinger Health System, Hershey, Pennsylvania

Christopher T. Ducko, MD
Senior Resident, Surgery, Pennsylvania State University; Penn State Geisinger Health System, Hershey, Pennsylvania

Frank W. Dupont, MD
Clinical Associate, Department of Anesthesia and Critical Care, University of Chicago, University of Chicago Hospitals, Chicago, Illinois

Fred H. Edwards, MD
Professor of Surgery, University of Florida; Chief, Adult Cardiothoracic Surgery, University of Florida Health Science Center, Jacksonville, Florida

M. Arisan Ergin, MD, PhD
Professor of Cardiothoracic Surgery, Mount Sinai School of Medicine, New York, New York

Jan D. Galla, MD, PhD
Assistant Professor of Cardiothoracic Surgery, Mount Sinai School of Medicine, New York, New York

Randall B. Griepp, MD
Professor of Cardiothoracic Surgery; Chairman, Department of Cardiothoracic Surgery, Mount Sinai School of Medicine, New York, New York

Frederick L. Grover, MD
Chief, Department of Surgery, University of Colorado Health Sciences Center, Denver, Colorado

Steven R. Gundry, MD
Professor and Head, Division of Cardiothoracic Surgery, Loma Linda University Medical Center, Loma Linda, California

Frank L. Hanley, MD
Professor of Surgery and Pediatric Cardiothoracic Surgeon, University of California, San Francisco

Alden H. Harken, MD
Professor and Chairman, Department of Surgery, University of Colorado Health Sciences Center; Chief of Surgery, University Hospital, Denver, Colorado

Jan Charles Horrow, MD
Clinical Professor, Anesthesiology, MCP Hahnemann University, Philadelphia; Vice President, Clinical Development, IBEX Technologies Corporation, Malvern, Pennsylvania

Christopher Komanapalli, BS
Medical Student, UCLA School of Medicine, Los Angeles, California

Hillel Laks, MD
Professor and Chief, Division of Cardiothoracic Surgery; Director, Heart and Heart–Lung Transplant Program, UCLA Medical Center, Los Angeles, California

Jonah Odim, MD, PhD
Assistant Professor of Surgery, Division of Cardiothoracic Surgery, UCLA School of Medicine, Los Angeles, California

Ed Petrossian, MD
Assistant Professor of Surgery, University of California, San Francisco; Pediatric Cardiothoracic Surgeon, Valley Children's Hospital, Madera, California

Benjamin J. Pomerantz, MD
Resident in Surgery, University of Colorado Health Sciences Center; University Hospital, Denver, Colorado

Hermann Reichenspurner, MD, PhD
Associate Professor, Department of Cardiothoracic Surgery, Ludwig-Maximilians Universitat, Klinikum Grosshadern, Munich, Germany

Fania L. Samuels, MD
Clinical Assistant Professor of Medicine, Division of Cardiology, MCP Hahnemann University; Staff, Department of Electrophysiology, Hahnemann University Hospital, Philadelphia, Pennsylvania

Louis E. Samuels, MD
Assistant Professor of Cardiothoracic Surgery, MCP Hahnemann University; Director of Clinical Research, Hahnemann University Hospital, Philadelphia, Pennsylvania

LeNardo D. Thompson, MD
Associate Professor of Surgery, University of California, San Franciso; Pediatric Cardiothoracic Surgeon, Oakland Children's Hospital, Oakland, California

Publisher's Preface

Andrew Wechsler, MD, is leaving the Editorial Board of *Advances in Cardiac Surgery*. Since the inception of the series 12 years ago, Dr Wechsler has been a formative and guiding influence on the philosophy and editorial content of what we believe is a highly successful annual publication in the field of cardiac surgery. Possessed of good humor and an insightful mind, Dr Wechsler has been of great value to his editorial colleagues and to the publishers of *Advances in Cardiac Surgery*, and we shall miss him.

Joining the Editorial Board will be Dr Bartley Griffith, who is professor of Surgery and chief of the Division of Cardiothoracic Surgery at the University of Pittsburgh. We welcome Dr Griffith, and we know that future volumes will undoubtedly benefit from his expertise.

Contents

C HAPTER 1

Cerebral Protection in Aortic Surgery*

Randall B. Griepp, MD
Professor of Cardiothoracic Surgery; Chairman, Department of
Cardiothoracic Surgery, Mount Sinai School of Medicine, New York,
New York

Jan D. Galla, MD, PhD
Assistant Professor of Cardiothoracic Surgery, Mount Sinai School of
Medicine, New York, New York

Anil Z. Apaydin, MD
Chief Resident in Cardiothoracic Surgery, Mount Sinai School of
Medicine, New York, New York

M. Arisan Ergin, MD, PhD
Professor of Cardiothoracic Surgery, Mount Sinai School of Medicine,
New York, New York

B rain injury following aortic surgery has, in recent years, gradually emerged as a cause of concern as complex aortic surgery has increasingly been performed for lesions in the ascending aorta, aortic arch, and proximal descending aorta that previously had been considered inoperable. With routine survival of patients after surgery requiring arrest of antegrade circulation to repair ascending aorta and arch aneurysms came enhanced expectations and the realization that survival was compromised in some of these patients by neurologic injury. The relatively high rate of cerebral sequelae after aortic surgery has prompted reassessment

---

*A version of this article was published as *Aortic Surgery and the Brain* in the proceedings of an international symposium on diseases of the aorta, called *Hot Topics in Aortic Diseases*, in São Paulo, Brazil in February 1999, sponsored by the Cardiovascular Surgery and Cardiology Division, Federal Division of São Paulo.

of the technique of hypothermic circulatory arrest (HCA), which is the mainstay of cerebral protection during aortic surgery, as well as a quest for ways of reducing the incidence of focal injury, the most frequent source of postoperative permanent neurologic disability.

MECHANISMS OF BRAIN INJURY

There are two major causes of permanent cerebral sequelae in these cases: embolization of particulate matter or air in sufficient quantity to permanently occlude cerebral vessels, and temporary oxygen deprivation for a duration long enough to cause early or delayed neuronal cell death. Unfortunately, the need to avoid both of these potential sources of cerebral injury often creates a conflict: for example, it is safest to manipulate and dissect an atheromatous arch under circulatory arrest, but this prolongs the total duration of cerebral ischemia. Thus, the minimization of cerebral injury during aortic surgery requires careful planning, constant vigilance, and ongoing judgments and decisions about the neurologic impact of various alternative maneuvers throughout the conduct of each procedure.

Whether the global component of brain injury after aortic surgery occurs during the ischemic interval or during reperfusion is not known, nor is the extent to which focal injury can be affected by management during reperfusion and early postoperatively. Possible mechanisms of injury during reperfusion after HCA include disturbances of cerebral blood flow, which have been documented in experimental animals and for which there is also some clinical evidence. Reactive hyperemia immediately on rewarming has been observed, followed by an inappropriate and sometimes very marked increase in cerebrovascular resistance lasting several hours postoperatively, which could result in compromised oxygen delivery especially in the presence of hemodynamic instability.[1-4] It has also been noted that cerebral edema occurs after HCA, and recent experiments in our laboratory have demonstrated that the increase in intracranial pressure that is seen after HCA can be mitigated by instituting an interval of cold reperfusion before rewarming, and by use of ultrafiltration.

Various agents have been postulated to contribute to the injury that may occur during reperfusion after an ischemic insult, including oxygen free radicals and excitotoxic amino acids.[5] Recently, it has been proposed that even injury that occurs during surgery may manifest itself only gradually postoperatively because it occurs by means of apoptosis, or programmed cell death, and thus may still be evolving during reperfusion and in the early postopertive period.

PHARMACOLOGY OF CEREBRAL PROTECTION

Pharmacologic strategies to combat the threats implicit in each hypothesis of how embolic and cerebral ischemic damage occurs during aortic surgery and its aftermath are appealing. Various different agents have been proposed, some have been tested experimentally, and a few have been used clinically. Barbiturates have been shown to provide some benefit in limiting the impact of ischemic injury in animal models, and have been used clinically in the hope of reducing cerebral sequelae from both focal and global injury.[5] In recent years, however, scrutiny has revealed that barbiturates may not add much protection to that of cerebral hypothermia if the hypothermia is sufficiently deep to abolish electrical activity in the brain. It has also been noted that doses of barbiturates sufficient to confer significant benefit in terms of cerebral protection result in myocardial depression, which may compromise cerebral blood flow during the so-called vulnerable period, when the susceptiblity of the brain to ischemia is heightened because of inappropriate cerebral vasoconstriction, and during which a reliably high cardiac output is therefore required.[1-4] Thus, many centers, including our own, no longer use barbiturates during aortic surgery.

The importance of cerebral edema after an ischemic insult has long been recognized, and steroids are almost universally used to combat this potential complication. They are often continued postoperatively in patients with prolonged cerebral ischemia.

Advocates of the use of free-radical scavengers postulate that some cerebral injury is occurring during reperfusion and can be prevented by these agents. Mannitol, in addition to reducing cerebral edema, is also a free-radical scavenger and is therefore doubly useful. Others have advocated the use of other free-radical scavengers such as superoxide dismutase.[5]

There is considerable experimental evidence implicating excitotoxic amino acids in some of the injury that occurs after prolonged HCA, showing that various kinds of excitotoxic amino acid receptor blocking agents are effective in reducing the extent of cerebral injury under these circumstances, as measured by behavioral recovery and histologic damage.[6-9] These studies implicate glutamate toxicity and perhaps a deficiency of nitric oxide in the pathogenesis of cerebral injury after prolonged HCA.[6,10,11] Thus far, unfortunately, none of the agents that are successful in mitigating cerebral injury experimentally is suitable for clinical use, but this avenue of pharmacologic inquiry seems promising.

The most recent potentially exciting hypothesis is that cerebral injury after aortic surgery occurs by the mechanism of apoptosis, or programmed cell death, a widespread normal homeostatic process that may be inappropriately triggered under these circumstances. There is already evidence that the steps involved in this pathway, which takes a number of hours to lead to irreversible injury, may be amenable to early interruption. This may open up a whole new way in which brain injury can be reduced pharmacologically. Some experimental evidence in animals has already shown reduction of infarct size after focal ischemia using specific inhibitors of the proteases involved in the apoptotic pathway, suggesting that some sublethally injured neurons may be rescued using this type of intervention.[12-18] But until further progress is made in discovering and testing pharmacologic means for cerebral protection, we must rely clinically on manipulation of temperature and use of selective cerebral perfusion strategies to protect the brain during aortic surgery. It is these strategies that will form the main emphasis of our discussion.

MONITORING FOR CEREBRAL INJURY

Because of the relative frequency of cerebral injury as a consequence of aortic surgery, and its often ominous prognosis, strategies for detecting possible damage intraoperatively are being sought increasingly, and ways of evaluating the success of cerebral electron protection both experimentally and clinically are becoming more sophisticated. Clinically, electroencephalographic (EEG) monitoring can be useful during cooling, especially for acute dissections in which cerebral malperfusion is a dreaded complication.[19] The EEG, however, is of somewhat limited utility when used in conjuction with deep hypothermia because the EEG signal disappears before sufficiently low temperatures for prolonged HCA are attained; cortical somatosensory evoked potential monitoring is somewhat more sensitive under these circumstances.[19] The sudden loss or disappearance of the EEG or somatosensory evoked potential can be very helpful in alerting the surgeon to an acute and possibly reversible technical problem intraoperatively, and a failure of electrical activity to recover appropriately during rewarming may also be useful for prognostication.

Clinical neurologic recovery after aortic surgery in most surgical series is assessed somewhat crudely, making it very difficult to evaluate the impact of differences in brain protection strategies unless the effects are dramatic. In addition, often the type or severity of injury in those patients who sustain significant neurologic damage is not specified. Less severe indications of possibly inadequate cerebral protection, such as delayed awakening, prolonged confusion, or deterioration of memory, are frequently not monitored, so that injury to the brain is only recognized if it is embolic, with focal manifestations, or if global, when very severe. Only a few studies have reported results of psychometric testing to try to detect more subtle global ischemic injury.[20-23]

In animal studies, the methodological problems involved in trying to evaluate brain protection are also often serious. Few studies report either histologic damage or behavioral evaluation. Many report various metabolic observations that cannot always reliably be correlated with neurologic outcome, usually without acknowledging that these observations are not, in fact, unequivocal evidence of brain injury or lack thereof. The presence of high levels of enzymes such as CPK-BB or S-100 protein in the cerebrospinal fluid or the circulation, patterns of recovery of cerebral blood flow and metabolism, and comparisons of various magnetic resonance assessments of intracellular pH or levels of energy stores are among the process variables that are dubious substitutes for evaluation of real outcome measures. Even the best assessments of cerebral outcome in animals, such as neurologic evaluation and cerebral histology, probably require greater damage to register an adverse outcome than is necessary to produce the cognitive changes that are a worrisome clinical consequence of aortic surgery.

USE OF HYPOTHERMIA FOR CEREBRAL PROTECTION

Two fundamental observations underpin the use of hypothermia for cerebral protection during aortic surgery: that cerebral circulation can be interrupted for short but significant intervals with eventual full recovery, and that cerebral metabolic rate decreases as temperature is lowered. Thus, at lower temperatures, longer intervals of cerebral oxygen deprivation are possible without significant sequelae.[24-26]

EXPERIMENTAL DATA

Quantification of the degree of metabolic suppression by lowering temperature is usually expressed as Q10: the degree of metabolic suppression seen with a 10°C difference in temperature. It is still unsettled whether the Q10 changes with increasingly deep hypothermia; some studies suggest that the rate as well as the degree of metabolic suppression may increase as hypothermia becomes more profound. Controversy arises because all Q10 measurements of cerebral metabolism depend on the methodology and assumptions used to calculate them. The major assumption is that a decrease in oxygen consumption reflects a physiologic autoregulatory reduction of the need for oxygen by neuronal cells rather than a dropout of dead neurons that are no longer capable of using oxygen. Tissue culture studies suggest that below 7°C to 8°C there is some form of cell injury related to loss of cell membrane fluidity that precludes a normal metabolic response to oxygen, so there may be a limit below which further lowering of temperature is no longer beneficial.[27,28]

We have measured cerebral oxygen metabolism in dog and pig under a wide range of temperatures using cerebral blood flow determined by the radioactive microsphere technique, and arteriovenous oxygen differences using samples from the carotid artery and sagittal sinus.[2,25,29-32] As shown in Figures 1 and 2, we have obtained consistent results over a range of hypothermic temperatures, suggesting a constant Q10 throughout the range of mild and deep hypothermia that is relevant clinically.[25,29]

In 37 patients in whom cerebral blood flow was estimated using a flow probe on the carotid artery, we found a Q10 of 2.3, which is in the same range as the Q10 found in our animal studies. With the assumption that circulatory arrest at 37°C can be tolerated safely for 5 minutes, this would predict the safe limits of circulatory arrest in humans to be as outlined in Table 1.[33]

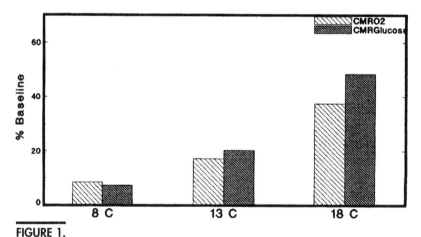

FIGURE 1.

Cerebral metabolic rates in weanling puppies after cooling to different temperatures. The rates of oxygen *(CMRO₂)* and glucose metabolism *(CMR Glucose)* at the end of the cooling interval were compared with baseline rates (at 37°C) for each experimental group. (Courtesy of Mezrow CK, Midulla PS, Sadeghi A, et al: Evaluation of cerebral metabolism and quantitative EEG following circulatory arrest and low flow cardiopulmonary bypass at different temperatures. *J Thorac Cardiovasc Surg* 107:1006-1019, 1994.)

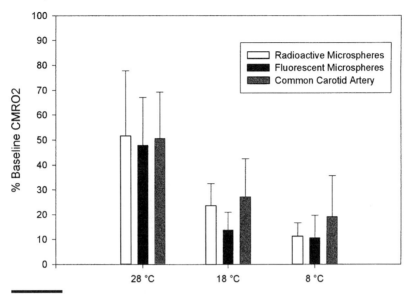

FIGURE 2.
Cerebral metabolic rates in pigs after cooling to different temperatures, as a percent of baseline measurements at 37°C. Calculations are based on three different methods of measuring cerebral blood flow. (Courtesy of Ehrlich MP, McCullough J, Juvonen T, et al: Effect of hypothermia on cerebral blood flow and metabolism in the pig. *Surgical Forum* 49:256-258, 1998.)

CLINICAL DATA

How can these data be reconciled with clinical experience, which suggests that durations of circulatory arrest up to 1 hour are usually safe at temperatures between 15°C and 20°C? To answer this question, we have undertaken several clinical studies of cerebral outcome in patients undergoing HCA.[20-23]

In the study by Ergin et al[20] in 1994, we found that 19% of patients exhibited what we call transient neurologic dysfunction (TND), consisting of symptoms present immediately after surgery that gradually improve, such as delayed awakening, prolonged agitation, confusion or disorientation, and Parkinson-like movements. A multivariate analysis showed that these symptoms correlate both with increasing age of the patients and with the duration of HCA. In patients with less that 30 minutes of HCA, the incidence of temporary dysfunction was 10% (Fig 3); it rose to 15% in patients with more than 40 minutes of HCA, was 30% in patients with 50 minutes of HCA, and was 60% if HCA lasted more than 1 hour.[20]

TABLE 1.
Projected Safe Duration of Hypothermic Circulatory Arrest at Different Temperatures

Temperature (°C)	Cerebral Metabolic Rate (% of Baseline)	Safe Duration of HCA (min)
37	100	5
30	56 (52-60)	9 (8-10)
25	37 (33-42)	14 (12-15)
20	24 (21-29)	21 (17-24)
15	16 (13-20)	31 (25-38)
10	11 (8-14)	45 (36-62)

Abbreviation: HCA, hypothermic circulatory arrest.

In a recent study by Reich et al,[23] patients underwent psychometric cognitive testing before and after surgery involving HCA at a temperature of 13°C. If HCA duration was 30 minutes or longer, patients had a significant postoperative decrease, compared with preoperative testing, in cognitive scores, whereas a decrease in postoperative function was not observed after intervals of HCA

Number of Patients

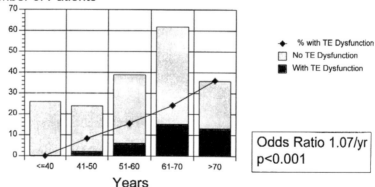

FIGURE 3.
Prevalence of temporary *(TE)* neurologic dysfunction in patients who underwent hypothermic circulatory arrest (HCA) as a function of duration of HCA. (Courtesy of Ergin MA, Galla JD, Lansman SE, et al: Hypothermic circulatory arrest in operations on the thoracic aorta: Determinants of operative mortality and neurologic outcome. *J Thorac Cardiovasc Surg* 107:788-799, 1994.)

less than 30 minutes. In an analysis on the same cohort of patients by Ergin et al,[22] there was a significant correlation between the occurrence of symptoms of TND and the persistence of impaired cognitive performance on psychometric testing 6 weeks after surgery. These data suggest that TND may not be a benign phenomenon but may be associated with prolonged, albeit subtle, cerebral injury.

CONCLUSIONS REGARDING HCA

From these data, we have concluded that 30 minutes is the limit for the safe duration of simple HCA.[22,23] We think that further metabolic suppression by more extreme lowering of the temperature may permit somewhat longer intervals, but there may be dangers associated with cooling below 7°C to 8°C.[28,34]

Certain aspects of the implementation of HCA are important to ensure its safety. Cooling must be thorough, which means that the interval of cooling should last at least 30 minutes.[35,36] Jugular bulb oxygen saturations should be measured before initiating arrest, and these saturations should exceed 95%; greater desaturation suggests too high a residual level of oxygen metabolism.[27,35-37] The level of hypothermia should be maintained during arrest by packing the head in ice.[38,39] Although some recent work suggests that, under special circumstances in the presence of congenital heart disease, a pH strategy of blood gas management during cooling is appropriate, alpha-stat blood gas management seems to be safer in adults.[40-44] Rapid rewarming should be avoided; there is some evidence to suggest that cold reperfusion may minimize reperfusion injury, and it seems prudent to restore cerebral metabolic demand slowly in view of a tendency toward cerebral vasoconstriction for several hours after HCA that may limit delivery of oxygen and preclude rapid metabolic recovery.[1-4]

ANTEGRADE CEREBRAL PERFUSION

The successful use of selective antegrade cerebral perfusion during aortic surgery is based on the fact that the brain is the organ most vulnerable to ischemia, and that adequate preservation of the other organs for surgically relevant intervals is adequately achieved by current methods of HCA.[5,45-48] In experimental studies, it is readily apparent that selective hypothermic antegrade perfusion provides much better cerebral protection than any other method, with much more rapid return of EEG and evoked potentials, better behavioral recovery, and virtual absence of cerebral histopathological lesions suggestive of ischemia even after prolonged intervals of arrest of systemic circulation.[2,25,30-32,38,39,46,49-51] Early experimental trials with normothermic or mildly hypothermic selective antegrade cerebral perfusion have been disappointing, so that only the combination of antegrade perfusion with deep hypothermia is appealing as an alternative to deep HCA alone.[52]

The necessary manipulation and cannulation of the cerebral vessels for selective antegrade cerebral perfusion can be difficult, however, and probably increases the likelihood of cerebral embolization, especially in older patients. Nevertheless, clinical experience with this technique, as reported by Bachet[53-55] and Kazui,[56,57] has been favorable.

Encouraged by these results, impressed by laboratory data demonstrating the superiority of selective antegrade perfusion, and sobered by experimental and clinical studies indicating the limitations of HCA alone, we have developed a technique for the use of selective antegrade cerebral perfusion when the interval of anticipated HCA is likely to be prolonged.[21,58] Our technique involves attachment of an island of arch vessels (with or without the left subclavian artery) to a 16-mm graft through which the arch vessels can be perfused. This can be accomplished from either a median sternotomy or a left thoracotomy approach and can usually be completed well within the 30 minutes we now consider safe for HCA alone. The remainder of the repair can be completed during antegrade perfusion through this graft; the perfusate is delivered at 10°C, at a flow rate regulated to achieve a radial artery pressure of 50 mm Hg. The final attachment of the graft to the cerebral vessels to the rest of the repair can easily be completed with an additional 8 to 10 minutes of HCA. This technique is now used in all cases of arch replacement and is illustrated in Figure 4.[58]

RETROGRADE CEREBRAL PERFUSION

Interest in the use of retrograde cerebral perfusion (RCP) was stimulated by the success of retrograde cardioplegia, and by its theoretical appeal not only as a possible way of enhancing cerebral protection during prolonged HCA, but also as a possible means of preventing embolic injury during aortic surgery.[49,59] Many enthusiastic clinical reports using this technique have been published in recent years, but on careful scrutiny it will be noted that the favorable outcomes achieved using RCP are often observed in patients with intervals of arrested circulation that would have resulted in a good outcome

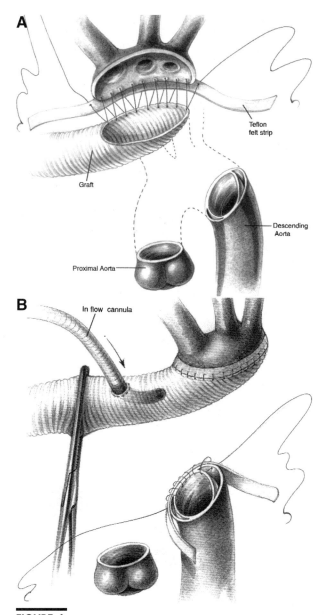

FIGURE 4.
Method for implementing selective hypothermic antegrade cerebral perfusion during operations requiring prolonged arrest of systemic circulation. **A,** A beveled 18-French Dacron graft is sutured to an island of aorta containing the cerebral vessels, using a Teflon felt strip, during hypothermic circulatory arrest (HCA). **B,** Selective antegrade cerebral perfusion is

(continued)

C

D

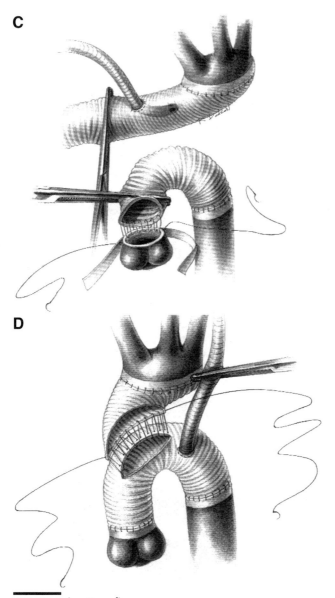

FIGURE 4. (continued)
instituted through the completed beveled graft to the cerebral vessels from
the perfusion circuit while the distal anastomosis is constructed. **C,** Once
the distal anastomosis has been completed, the proximal anastomoses can
be carried out while antegrade perfusion of the distal lower body is provided by a second perfusion catheter inserted into the graft (seen in **D**),
while selective cerebral perfusion continues uninterrupted through a

(continued)

E

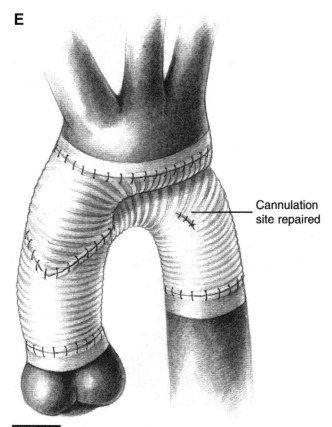

Cannulation
site repaired

FIGURE 4. (continued)
separate cannula. **D,** During another brief period of HCA, the aortic arch
reconstruction and the cerebral vessel graft are sutured to one another. **E,**
The completed aortic arch reconstruction, with the distal perfusion cannulation site repaired. (Courtesy of Galla JD, McCullough JN, Griepp RB:
Aortic arch replacement for dissection. *Operative Techniques Thorac
Cardiovasc Surg* 4:58-76, 1999.)

using HCA alone.[60-74] Furthermore, these studies often use histor-
ical controls, and none has involved careful assessment of neurologic outcome using psychometric testing.

Unfortunately, laboratory investigations of RCP have been complicated by the unsuitability of the dog for such studies, requiring
use of retrograde perfusion techniques in the laboratory that may
have little clinical relevance. Attempts to draw conclusions from
comparisons of experiments involving various other species with
significant differences in their anatomy from one another and

from the cerebral circulation of humans are often frustrating, especially because there are also major differences among studies in other technical aspects of retrograde perfusion, including pressures and flow rates, and whether major collateral vessels, such as the inferior vena cava (IVC), are occluded during retrograde perfusion.[1,30,39,50,75-85] This has resulted in widely diverging assessments of both the utility and safety of RCP.

The most striking observation, made in several experimental studies, is how little of the retrograde flow actually goes to the brain; most of the flow is shunted via the azygous system to the IVC, although a small amount clearly reaches the brain via collaterals surrounding the spinal cord.[76] Our observations, based on aortic arch return measured during retrograde flow into the superior vena cava (SVC) in a porcine model, suggest that less than 5% of retrograde flow traverses the cerebral circulation.[39,50] This is too little to sustain metabolic needs over a prolonged interval even in the presence of hypothermia, but clearly some uptake of oxygen and nutrients does occur during RCP. The decline in intracellular pH seen during arrest of antegrade circulation has been shown to be less severe with RCP than with HCA alone, and use of RCP results in a slightly more favorable outcome histologically than HCA, even when the head is packed in ice.[39,50,84-86] Under some circumstances, part of the benefit of RCP may be from improved cooling. In addition, RCP may remove potentially toxic metabolites from the cerebral circulation—metabolites that would otherwise accumulate during HCA and reduce brain injury during reperfusion.

Unfortunately, RCP is also associated with the development of cerebral edema to an extent greater than that seen with HCA, becoming even more severe with longer durations of RCP. Maneuvers that increase the effectiveness of retrograde perfusion usually also increase the rate at which cerebral edema accumulates, and cerebral edema appears to contribute to the cerebral histopathology that is sometimes seen after prolonged HCA utilizing RCP.[50,77,87]

Even though experimental studies have failed to show that use of RCP bestows an unequivocal advantage by enhancing protection during prolonged HCA, RCP has been enthusiastically adopted by many centers.[34,60-63,65-74] Its use is especially appealing for short intervals to reduce the risk of embolization of atherosclerotic debris into the arch vessels during surgery. We use it in patients who have had clot or atheroma in the aorta identified either preoperatively or intraoperatively. We infuse into either one or both vena cavae at a flow rate of 800 to 1000 mL/min initially, and then lower the rate to 100 to 500 mL/min as required to generate a pressure of 15 to 20 mm Hg in the SVC.[21,46]

PREVENTION OF CEREBRAL EMBOLI

Prevention of emboli is not a major concern in younger patients undergoing a Bentall procedure or in most patients undergoing operation for type A dissection. For older patients, however, the presence of clot or atheroma in the aortic lumen is emerging as a major risk factor for mortality and cerebral injury.

The predominant risk occurs with manipulation of the aorta and dislodgment of debris by cannulation and altered flow within the aorta. Therefore, it is vital to avoid manipulating an aorta containing clot or atheroma upstream of the cerebral vessels—in the ascending aorta or arch when perfusing antegrade, and in the descending aorta when perfusion is via the femoral artery. It is also important to cannulate away from the cerebral vessels to avoid dislodging clot or atheroma as a result of turbulence near the tip of the perfusion catheter. The femoral artery and, more recently, the subclavian artery are therefore becoming the cannulation sites of choice in high-risk patients. Avoidance of clamps near the cerebral vessels is also recommended because of the danger of dislodging debris that can embolize. In the descending aorta, it is imperative to avoid clamping within 2 to 3 cm distal to the left subclavian, and in the ascending aorta and arch, the clamp should be placed away from the innominate artery.

In addition, careful cleansing of any retained vessel walls is important. The wall should be wiped with gauze, but flushing with saline, which may carry debris into the cerebral vessels, should be avoided. Careful and repeated aspiration of the orifice of each retained vessel should be carried out after opening the aorta and after debridement of the adjacent arch. We do not believe that air trapping in open arch vessels is a significant problem, and so we repeatedly gently aspirate these vessels. Care is taken to remove all air before restoring perfusion, however, and a brief period of retrograde perfusion may be used to de-air as well as to enhance cleansing by aspiration. We also try to ensure that air embolism does not occur from the heart.

CURRENT PROTOCOL FOR BRAIN PROTECTION

The likelihood of finding clot or atheroma in the aorta is predicted preoperatively by considering the patient's age, any evidence of atherosclerosis in peripheral vessels, and by reviewing the CT scan or MRI; the risk of embolism is also assessed intraoperatively by transesophageal echocardiography. In young patients with evidence of aortic debris, femoral artery cannulation is recommended, but subclavian artery cannulation is preferred in all other high-risk patients. If the approach is via a median sternotomy, the right subclavian artery should be used; the left subclavian can be cannulated from within the chest through a left thoracotomy incision. Perfusion should be instituted gradually to minimize the chance of dislodging potential emboli.

Cooling should be carried out for at least 30 minutes and continued until the jugular venous saturation, which should be measured repeatedly, exceeds 95%. If a significant period of circulatory arrest is likely to be required, cooling should be continued to a temperature of 10°C to 13°C, with a blood temperature of 10°C. The head should be packed in ice. Manipulation of any questionable segments of the aorta should be avoided. Once circulatory arrest has been achieved, dissection of a distal cuff or island of cerebral vessels should be done open, as well as debridement of loose atheroma from any retained vessel wall. Each of the arch vessels should carefully be aspirated. If excessive debris is present, a brief period of retrograde perfusion with an SVC pressure between 15 and 20 mm Hg should be used. The total duration of circulatory arrest should be limited to less than 30 minutes. An island of cerebral vessels should be perfused antegrade via the graft or the subclavian artery if the procedure is anticipated to be prolonged. Separate grafts should be anastomosed to one another with a brief period of HCA after all other reconstruction has been completed.

Warming should be gradual, with a maximal gradient of 10°C between the blood and the esophageal temperature. Partial bypass with pulsatile perfusion and the heart well resuscitated should be carried out for about 30 minutes. From a temperature of 10°C to 12°C, 50 to 60 minutes of rewarming will be necessary. At an esophageal temperature of 35°C to 36°C, cardiopulmonary bypass is discontinued; rectal temperature at this time is likely to be 30°C to 32°C. The patient is then allowed to warm slowly over a period of several hours in the intensive care unit.

Methylprednisolone (1 g) is given at the time of starting cardiopulmonary bypass in all aortic surgery patients. If the total duration of HCA exceeds 30 minutes, an additional 1.5 g of methylprednisolone is given over a 48-hour period after surgery.

SURGICAL RESULTS

Since 1992, 225 patients have undergone aortic surgery, with an overall mortality rate of 7%. Of 141 patients who were considered at high risk of neurologic complications because of age exceeding 60 years or evidence of clot or atheroma within the aorta, the mortality rate was 6%. Permanent neurologic dysfunction occurred in 8% of patients overall, and in 10% of patients in the high-risk group. We think that our management of these patients is gradually improving, with a lower incidence of neurologic complications in the most recent cohort of patients.

In the last few years, we have made great progress in identifying the patients most at risk for neurologic complications, and modifying our procedures to minimize cerebral injury. Further progress is most likely to arise from improved understanding of the pathogenesis of cerebral injury after HCA and focal ischemia, which should lead to the development of improved neuroprotective strategies. At present, the inhibition of glutamate receptors and interference with early steps involved in apoptosis appear to be the most promising pharmacologic approaches for future improvements in cerebral protection during aortic surgery.

REFERENCES

1. Jonassen AE, Quaegebeur JM, Young WL: Cerebral blood flow velocity in pediatric patients is reduced after cardiopulmonary bypass with profound hypothermia. *J Thorac Cardiovasc Surg* 110:934-943, 1995.
2. Mezrow CK, Midulla PS, Sadeghi A, et al: A vulnerable interval for cerebral injury: Comparison of hypothermic circulatory arrest and low flow cardiopulmonary bypass. *Cardiol Young* 3:287-298, 1993.
3. O'Hare B, Bissonnette B, Bohn D, et al: Persistent low cerebral blood flow velocity following profound hypothermic circulatory arrest in infants. *Can J Anaesth* 42:964-971, 1995.
4. van der Linden J: Cerebral hemodynamics after low-flow versus no-flow procedures. *Ann Thorac Surg* 59:1321-1325, 1995.
5. Griepp EB, Griepp RB: Cerebral consequences of hypothermic circulatory arrest in adults. *J Card Surg* 134-155, 1992.
6. Baumgartner WA, Walinsky P, Salazar JD, et al: Assessing the impact of cerebral injury after cardiac surgery: Will determining the mechanism reduce this injury? *Ann Thorac Surg* 67:1871-1873, 1999.
7. Redmond JM, Zehr KJ, Blue ME, et al: AMPA glutamate receptor antagonism reduces neurologic injury after hypothermic circulatory arrest. *Ann Thorac Surg* 59:579-584, 1995.
8. Redmond JM, Gillinov AM, Blue ME, et al: The monoganglioside, GM1, reduces neurologic injury associated with hypothermic circulatory arrest. *Surgery* 114:324-333, 1993.
9. Redmond JM, Gillinov AM, Zehr KJ, et al: Glutamate excitotoxicity: A mechanism of neurologic injury associated with hypothermic circulatory arrest. *J Thorac Cardiovasc Surg* 107:776-787, 1994.
10. Hiramatsu T, Jonas RA, Miura T, et al: Cerebral metabolic recovery

from deep hypothermic circulatory arrest after treatment with arginine and nitro-arginine methyl ester. *J Thorac Cardiovasc Surg* 112:698-707, 1996.

11. Tsui SSL, Kirshbom PM, Davies MJ, et al: Nitric oxide production affects cerebral perfusion and metabolism after deep hypothermic ciruclatory arrest. *Ann Thorac Surg* 61:1699-1707, 1996.

12. Chen J, Nagayama T, Jin K, et al: Induction of caspase-3–like protease may mediate delayed neuronal death in the hippocampus after transient cerebral ischemia. *J Neurosci* 18:4914-4928, 1998.

13. Cheng Y, Deshmukh M, D'Costa A, et al: Caspase inhibitor affords neuroprotection with delayed administration in a rat model of neonatal hypoxic-ischemic brain injury. *J Clin Invest* 101:1992-1999, 1998.

14. Endres M, Namura S, Shimizu-Sasamata M, et al: Attenuation of delayed neuronal death by inhibition of the caspase family. *J Cereb Blood Flow Metab* 18:238-247, 1998.

15. Ferrari G, Greene LA: Prevention of apoptotic death by neurotrophic agents and ganglioside GM1: Insights and speculations regarding a common mechanism. *Perspect Dev Neurobiol* 3:93-100, 1996.

16. Hara H, Friedlander RM, Gagliardini V, et al: Inhibition of interleukin 1B converting family enzyme family proteases reduces ischemic and excitotoxic neuronal damage. *Proc Natl Acad Sci U S A* 94:2007-2012, 1997.

17. Namura S, Zhu J, Fink K, et al: Activation and cleavage of caspase-3 in apoptosis induced by experimental cerebral ischemia. *J Neurosci* 18:3659-3668, 1998.

18. Rosenbaum DM, D'Amore J, Llena J, et al: Pretreatment with intraventricular aurintricarboxylic acid decreases infarct size by inhibiting apoptosis following transient global ischemia in gerbils. *Ann Neurol* 43:654-660, 1998.

19. Ghariani S, Liard L, Spaey J, et al: Retrospective study of somatosensory evoked potential monitoring in deep hypothermic circulatory arrest. *Ann Thorac Surg* 67:1915-1918, 1999.

20. Ergin MA, Galla JD, Lansman SE, et al: Hypothermic circulatory arrest in operations on the thoracic aorta: Determinants of operative mortality and neurologic outcome. *J Thorac Cardiovasc Surg* 107:788-799, 1994.

21. Ergin MA, Griepp EB, Lansman SL, et al: Hypothermic circulatory arrest and other methods of cerebral protection during operations on the thoracic aorta. *J Card Surg* 9:525-537, 1994.

22. Ergin MA, Uysal S, Reich DL, et al: Temporary neurologic dysfunction following deep hypothermic circulatory arrest: A clinical marker of long-term functional deficit. *Ann Thorac Surg* 67:1887-1890, 1999.

23. Reich DL, Uysal S, Sliwinski M, et al: Neuropsychologic outcome after deep hypothermic circulatory arrest in adults. *J Thorac Cardiovasc Surg* 117:156-163, 1999.

24. Gillinov AM, Redmond JM, Zehr KJ, et al: Superior cerebral protection with profound hypothermia during circulatory arrest. *Ann Thorac Surg* 55:1432-1439, 1993.

25. Mezrow CK, Midulla PS, Sadeghi A, et al: Evaluation of cerebral metabolism and quantitative EEG following circulatory arrest and low flow cardiopulmonary bypass at different temperatures. *J Thorac Cardiovasc Surg* 107:1006-1019, 1994.

26. O'Connor JV, Wilding T, Farmer P, et al: The protective effect of profound hypothermia on the canine central nervous system during one hour of circulatory arrest. *Ann Thorac Surg* 41:225-259, 1986.

27. Kurth CD, O'Rourke MM, O'Hara IB: Comparison of pH stat and alpha-stat cardiopulmonary bypass on cerebral oxygenation and blood flow in relation to hypothermic circulatory arrest in piglets. *Anesthesiology* 89:110-118, 1998.

28. Kruuv J, Lepock JR: Factors influencing survival of mammalian cells exposed to hypothermia. *Cryobiology* 32:191-198, 1995.

29. Ehrlich MP, McCullough J, Juvonen T, et al: Effect of hypothermia on cerebral blood flow and metabolism in the pig. *Surgical Forum* 49:256-258, 1998.

30. Mezrow CK, Sadeghi AM, Gandsas A, et al: Cerebral blood flow and metabolism in hypothermic circulatory arrest. *Ann Thorac Surg* 54:609-616, 1992.

31. Mezrow CK, Gandsas A, Sadeghi AM, et al: Metabolic correlates of neurologic and behavioral injury after prolonged hypothermic circulatory arrest. *J Thorac Cardiovasc Surg* 109:959-975, 1995.

32. Mezrow CK, Sadeghi A, Gandsas A, et al: Cerebral effects of low flow cardiopulmonary bypass and hypothermic circulatory arrest. *Ann Thorac Surg* 57:532-539, 1994.

33. McCullough JN, Zhang N, Reich D, et al: Cerebral metabolic suppression during circulatory arrest in humans. *Ann Thorac Surg* 67:1895-1899, 1999.

34. Kruuv J, Glofcheski DJ, Lepock JR: Evidence for two modes of hypothermic damage in five cell lines. *Cryobiology* 32:182-190, 1995.

35. Greeley WJ, Kern FH, Ungerleider RM, et al: The effect of hypothermic cardiopulmonary bypass and total circulatory arrest on cerebral metabolism in neonates, infants and children. *J Thorac Cardiovasc Surg* 101:783-794, 1991.

36. Kern FH, Ungerleider RM, Schulman SR, et al: Comparing two strategies of cardiopulmonary bypass cooling on jugular venous oxygen saturation in neonates and infants. *Ann Thorac Surg* 60:1198-1202, 1995.

37. Kirshbom, PM, Skaryak LR, DIBernardo LR, et al: pH-stat cooling improves cerebral metabolic recovery after circulatory arrest in a piglet model of aortopulmonary collaterals. *J Thorac Cardiovasc Surg* 111:147-157, 1996.

38. Crittenden MD, Roberts CS, Rosa L, et al: Brain protection during circulatory arrest. *Ann Thorac Surg* 51:942-947 1991.

39. Midulla PS, Gandsas A, Sadeghi AM, et al: Comparison of retrograde cerebral perfusion to antegrade cerebral perfusion and hypothermic circulatory arrest in a chronic porcine model. *J Card Surg* 9:560-575, 1994.

40. duPlessis AJ, Jonas RA, Wypij D, et al: Perioperative effects of alpha-stat versus pH-stat strategies for deep hypothermic cardiopulmonary bypass in infants. *J Thorac Cardiovasc Surg* 114:991-1000, 1997.

41. Hiramatsu T, Miura T, Forbess JM, et al: pH strategies and cerebral energetics before and after circulatory arrest. *J Thorac Cardiovasc Surg* 109:948-958, 1995.

42. Jonas RA, Bellinger DC, Rappaport LA, et al: Relation of pH strategy and developmental outcome after hypothermic circulatory arrest. *J Thorac Cardiovasc Surg* 106:362-368, 1993.

43. Murkin JM: Anesthesia, the brain, and cardiopulmonary bypass. *Ann Thorac Surg* 56:1461-1463, 1993.

44. Wong PC, Barlow CF, Hickey PR, et al: Factors associated with choreoathetosis after cardiopulmonary bypass in children with congenital heart disease. *Circulation* 86:II-118-126, 1992.

45. Ergin MA, O'Connor J, Guinto R, et al: Experience with profound hypothermia and circulatory arrest in the treatment of aneurysms of the aortic arch: Aortic arch replacement for acute arch dissections. *J Thorac Cardiovasc Surg* 84:649-655, 1982.

46. Griepp RB, Juvonen T, Griepp EB, et al: Is retrograde cerebral perfusion an effective means of neural support during deep hypothermic circulatory arrest? *Ann Thorac Surg* 64:913-916, 1997.

47. Lansman SL, Griepp RB: Resection of aortic arch aneurysms using hypothermic circulatory arrest, in Kaiser LR, Kron IL, Spray TL (eds): *Mastery of Cardiothoracic Surgery.* Lippincott-Raven, 1998, pp 472-478.

48. Svennson LG, Crawford ES, Hess KR, et al: Deep hypothermia with circulatory arrest: Determinants of stroke and mortality in 656 patients. *J Thorac Cardiovasc Surg*; 106:19-31, 1993.

49. Juvonen T, Weisz DJ, Wolfe D, et al: Can retrograde perfusion mitigate cerebral injury after particulate embolization? A study in a chronic porcine model. *J Thorac Cardiovasc Surg* 115:1142-1159, 1998.

50. Juvonen T, Zhang N, Wolfe D, et al: Retrograde cerebral perfusion enhances cerebral protection during prolonged hypothermic circulatory arrest: A study in a chronic porcine model. *Ann Thorac Surg* 66:38-50, 1998.

51. Mezrow CK, Midulla PS, Sadeghi AM, et al: Quantitative electroencephalography: A method to assess cerebral injury after hypothermic circulatory arrest. *J Thorac Cardiovasc Surg* 109:925-934, 1995.

52. Cook DJ, Oliver WC, Orszulak TA, et al: Cardiopulmonary bypass temperature, hematocrit and cerebral oxygen delivery in humans. *Ann Thorac Surg* 60:1671-1677, 1995.

53. Bachet J, Guilmet D, Goudot B, et al: Antegrade cerebral perfusion with cold blood: A 13-year experience. *Ann Thorac Surg* 67:1874-1878, 1999.

54. Bachet J, Guilmet D, Goudot B, et al: Cold cerebroplegia: A new technique of cerebral protection during operations on the transverse aortic arch. *J Thorac Cardiovasc Surg* 102:85-94, 1991.

55. Bachet J, Goudot B, Droyfus G, et al: Antegrade selective cerebral per-

fusion with cold blood during aortic arch surgery. *J Card Surg* 12:193-200, 1997.

56. Kazui T, Kimura N, Yamada O, et al: Surgical outcome of aortic arch aneurysm using selective cerebral perfusion. *Ann Thorac Surg* 57:904-911, 1994.

57. Sakurada T, Kazui T, Tanaka H, et al: Comparative experimental study of cerebral protection during aortic arch reconstruction. *Ann Thorac Surg* 61:1348-1354, 1996.

58. Galla JD, McCullough JN, Griepp RB: Aortic arch replacement for dissection. *Op Tech Thorac Cardiovasc Surg* 4:58-76, 1999.

59. Yerlioglu ME, Wolfe D, Mezrow CK, et al: The effect of retrograde cerebral perfusion after particulate embolization to the brain. *J Thorac Cardiovasc Surg* 110:1470-1485, 1995.

60. Bavaria JE, Woo J, Hall RA, et al: Retrograde cerebral and distal aortic perfusion during ascending and thoracoabdominal aortic operations. *Ann Thorac Surg* 60:345-353, 1995.

61. Coselli JS: Retrograde cerebral perfusion via a superior vena cava cannula for aortic arch aneurysm operations. *Ann Thorac Surg* 57:1668-1669, 1994.

62. Coselli JS, Buket S, Djukanovic B: Aortic arch operation: Current treatment and results. *Ann Thorac Surg* 59:19-27, 1995.

63. Kitamura M, Hashimoto A, Akimoto T, et al: Operation for type A dissection: Introduction of retrograde cerebral perfusion. *Ann Thorac Surg* 59:1195-1199, 1995.

64. Levy WJ, Levin SK, Bavaria JE: Cerebral oxygenation during retrograde perfusion. *Ann Thorac Surg* 60:184-186, 1995.

65. Lin PJ, Chang JP, Tan PCP, et al: Protection of the brain by retrograde cerebral perfusion during circulatory arrest. *J Thorac Cardiovasc Surg* 108:969-974, 1994.

66. Lin PJ, Chang CH, Tan PPC, et al: Prolonged circulatory arrest in moderate hypothermia with retrograde cerebral perfusion: Is brain ischemic? *Circulation* 94:II-169-172, 1996.

67. Lytle BW, McCarthy PM, Meaney KM, et al: Systemic hypothermia and circulatory arrest combined with arterial perfusion of the superior vena cava: Effective intraoperative cerebral protection. *J Thorac Cardiovasc Surg* 109:738-743, 1995.

68. McLoughlin TM, Carter WC, King CD: Continuous retrograde cerebral perfusion as an adjunct to brain protection during deep hypothermic systemic circulatory arrest. *J Cardiothorac Vasc Anesth* 9:205-214, 1995.

69. Moshkovitz Y, David T, Caleb M, et al: Circulatory arrest under moderate systemic hypothermia and cold retrograde cerebral perfusion. *Ann Thorac Surg* 66:1179-1184, 1998.

70. Pagano D, Carey JA, Patel RL, et al: Retrograde cerebral perfusion: Clinical experience in emergency and elective aortic operations. *Ann Thorac Surg* 59:393-397, 1995.

71. Safi HJ, Brien HW, Winter JN, et al: Brain protection via cerebral ret-

rograde perfusion during aortic arch aneurysm repair. *Ann Thorac Surg* 56:270-276, 1993.

72. Ueda Y, Miki S, Kusuhara K, et al: Deep hypothermic systemic circulatory arrest and continuous retrograde cerebral perfusion for surgery of aortic arch aneurysms. *Eur J Cardiothorac Surg* 6:36-41, 1992.

73. Usui A, Abe T, Murase M: Early clinical results of retrograde cerebral perfusion for aortic arch operations in Japan. *Ann Thorac Surg* 62:94-104, 1996.

74. Usui A, Hotta T, Hiroura M, et al: Retrograde cerebral perfusion through a superior vena caval cannula protects the brain. *Ann Thorac Surg* 53:47-53, 1992.

75. Boeckxstaens CJ, Flameng WJ: Retrograde cerebral perfusion does not perfuse the brain in nonhuman primates. *Ann Thorac Surg* 60:319-328, 1995.

76. deBrux JL, Subayi JB, Pegis JD, et al: Retrograde cerebral perfusion: Anatomic study of the distribution of blood to the brain. *Ann Thorac Surg* 60:1294-1298, 1995.

77. Nojima T, Magara T, Nakajima Y, et al: Optimal perfusion pressure for experimental retrograde cerebral perfusion. *J Card Surg* 9:548-559, 1994.

78. Nojima T, Nakajima Y: Experimental retrograde cerebral perfusion via bilateral maxillary vein in dogs. *Ann Thorac Surg* 61:1289-1291, 1996.

79. Oohara K, Usui A, Tanaka M, et al: Determination of organ blood flows during retrograde inferior vena caval perfusion. *Ann Thorac Surg* 58:139-145, 1994.

80. Pagano D, Boivin CM, Faroqui MH, et al: Retrograde perfusion through the superior vena cava perfuses the brain in human beings. *J Thorac Cardiovasc Surg* 111:270-272, 1996.

81. Safi HJ, Iliopoulos DC, Gopinath SR, et al: Retrograde cerebral perfusion during profound hypothermia and circulatory arrest in pigs. *Ann Thorac Surg* 59:1107-1112, 1995.

82. Usui A, Oohara K, Liu T, et al: Comparative experimental study between retrograde cerebral perfusion and circulatory arrest. *J Thorac Cardiovasc Surg* 107:1228-1236, 1994.

83. Usui A, Oohara K, Liu T, et al: Determination of optimum retrograde cerebral perfusion conditions. *J Thorac Cardiovasc Surg* 107:300-308, 1994.

84. Watanabe T, Iijima Y, Abe K, et al: Retrograde brain perfusion beyond the venous valves: Hemodynamic and intracellular pH mapping. *J Thorac Cardiovasc Surg* 111:36-44, 1996.

85. Ye J, Yang L, DelBigio MR, et al: Neuronal damage after hypothermic circulatory arrest and retrograde cerebral perfusion in the pig. *Ann Thorac Surg* 61:1316-1322, 1996.

86. Saiutou H, Watanabe T, Zhang JW, et al: Regional tissue blood flow and pH in the brain during deep hypothermic retrograde brain perfusion. *J Surg Res* 72:135-140, 1997.

87. Yoshimura N, Okada M, Ota T, et al: Pharmacologic intervention for ischemic brain edema after retrograde cerebral perfusion. *J Thorac Cardiovasc Surg* 109:1173-1181, 1995.

CHAPTER 2

Ischemia and the Myocardium

Benjamin J. Pomerantz, MD
Resident in Surgery, University of Colorado Health Sciences Center;
University Hospital, Denver, Colorado

Alden H. Harken, MD
Professor and Chairman, Department of Surgery, University of Colorado
Health Sciences Center; Chief of Surgery, University Hospital, Denver,
Colorado

Reduction in myocardial blood flow is no longer thought to solely produce irreversible myocardial damage, but rather it induces a spectrum of cell signals leading to both protective and destructive clinical syndromes. A brief period of transient ischemia before a prolonged ischemic insult results in cardioprotection. Conversely, prolonged (unprotected) myocardial ischemia inflicts cell death (apoptosis and necrosis). As the mechanisms responsible for these ischemic syndromes are elucidated, numerous new therapies have evolved targeting specific signaling steps. Each therapy persuasively promises improvement in clinical outcome of myocardial ischemia. This chapter will explore the response of the myocardium to ischemia (Fig 1), discuss methods of inducing protection (preconditioning) against ischemia, examine the cellular signals activated by ischemia, and offer some clinically accessible strategies to protect the myocardium from the myocellular damage associated with ischemia.

PRECONDITIONING

Myocardium exposed to a brief period (several minutes) of "transient" ischemia before a prolonged period of ischemia (as much as an hour) is protected against the prolonged ischemic challenge.

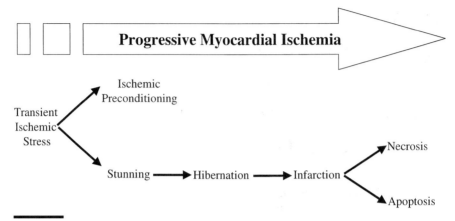

FIGURE 1.
Spectrum of the myocardial responses to ischemia.

This paradoxical response to brief ischemia has been termed "ischemic preconditioning" (IPC).[1] Ischemic preconditioning did not altogether prevent necrosis, but rather it altered the pattern of myocardial damage.[1] Necrosis in preconditioned myocardium was patchy with normal myocytes interspersed within areas of muscle damage, whereas nonpreconditioned hearts exhibit confluent necrosis.[1]

IPC has been demonstrated in the clinical setting. Angina before a myocardial infarction may paradoxically serve as a constructive preconditioning stimulus. The Thrombolysis in Myocardial Infarction (TIMI) 4 trial confirmed a protective effect of angina before myocardial infarction.[2] Patients with antecedent angina were less likely to develop congestive heart failure or shock and had a smaller area of infarction as indicated by creatine kinase release. In addition, the patients with preceding angina were less likely to evolve Q waves or have in-hospital deaths. These investigators concluded that antecedent angina conferred a measurable clinical benefit resulting from IPC. Patients undergoing percutaneous transluminal angioplasty have been a focus of the clinical application of IPC. The ability to favorably precondition myocardium using transient coronary occlusion before angioplasty has been reported.[3-7] IPC has also been accomplished in patients on cardiopulmonary bypass by intermittent cross clamping of the aorta before a sustained cross clamping.[8] These surgical patients treated with IPC exhibited increased tissue adenosine triphosphate (ATP) levels and decreased troponin T release.

Preconditioning can be divided into both acute and delayed phases. Acute, or early, preconditioning describes the delay of infarction as a result of one or more proceeding cycles of ischemia and reperfusion. Acute preconditioning evolves immediately. Delayed, or late, preconditioning describes an effect that requires 12 to 72 hours to be established.[9,10] We have reported that early preconditioning involves the upregulation of already existing receptor-mediated pathways.[11-16] We[17] and others[9] have observed that the late phase of preconditioning obligates new protein synthesis. The effectors that have been implicated in IPC include adenosine, acetylcholine, protein kinase C (PKC), bradykinin, and catecholamines.

A complex cascade of events including PKC activation,[18,19] phospholipase C, diacylglycerol, and G-protein activation occurs after the initial preconditioning stimulus. Recently a large body of evidence has been produced implicating the mitochondrial K_{ATP} channel as the final common effector of acute preconditioning. Cardioprotection can be achieved with $MitoK_{ATP}$ channel openers (diazoxide and pinacidil).[20-22] Pharmacologic blockade of the $MitoK_{ATP}$ channel with selective and nonselective blockers (5-hydroxydeconate and glyburide) inhibits both pharmacologic and ischemic preconditioning.[21,23-25] We have documented this preconditioning mechanism in human myocardium.[26] We also note the apparent relevance of this observation to patients with diabetes. Oral sulfonylurea hypoglycemic agents (glyburide) prevent IPC and may account for the paradoxically increased cardiovascular mortality of diabetic patients controlled with oral agents as opposed to insulin.[23]

In addition to ischemia, multiple clinically accessible pharmacologic agents serve as preconditioning stimuli. Adenosine acts as a preconditioning stimulus in human myocardium through PKC and K_{ATP} channel activation.[23,25-27]

IPC, along with adenosine and norepinephrine, leads to elevation in intracellular Ca^{2+}.[11,28,29] The role of calcium in preconditioning has been demonstrated by blockade of the L-type calcium channel with resultant attenuation of protective preconditioning.[29] Increasing the calcium concentration within the myocyte before an ischemic insult leads to constructive preconditioning in multiple species.[29-31]

PKC appears to be involved in preconditioning as well. Multiple forms of PKC exist within the myocardium. PKC isoforms appear to act distally within the preconditioning cascade. Previous work from our laboratory[31-36] and others[29,37] has demonstrated the obligate role of PKC in preconditioning. Each isoform of PKC plays a separate role in myocardial preconditioning. Experimental activation and blockade of specific isoforms have enabled investigations of each PKC isoform.[11,16,35,36] PKC isoforms η and δ are responsible for functional and viability protection, respectively.[13,14,35] Ischemic, endogenous, and exogenous stimuli all activate PKC.[11,29,30,37-39]

Delayed preconditioning represents subacute adaptation of the myocardium to ischemia.[9] This form of preconditioning represents the second effect of preconditioning and begins at a minimum of 12 hours and may extend up to 3 days.[40] Effects of delayed preconditioning include antiarrhythmic protection and resistance to myocardial stunning.[41,42] Delayed preconditioning and acute preconditioning share many features including initiators and intracellular signals. A central mediator of delayed preconditioning is also activated PKC.[43] If the action of PKC is blocked with pharmacologic agents, the beneficial effects of delayed preconditioning are abolished.[43]

Some progress has been made in delineating the mechanisms by which ischemic or pharmacologic preconditioning functions to protect the myocardium for a subsequent ischemic challenge. Myocardial ATP levels are increased, tumor necrosis factor (TNF)-α levels decrease, nitric oxide (NO) production increases, and leukocyte superoxide production decreases as a result of a preconditioning stimulus. It is likely that these events conspire to improve function and decrease myocardial damage in preconditioned myocardium both through the attenuation of myocellular inflammation and through the enhancement of cardiac bioenergetic status.

Delayed preconditioning involves obligate protein synthesis. These protective proteins include a family of heat shock proteins, inducible NO synthase (iNOS), catalase, and superoxide dismutase (SOD).[31] Heat shock proteins protect the heart by decreasing TNF and interleukin (IL)-1 production through interaction with nuclear factor kappa B (NFκB). By preventing activation of the transcriptional regulator (NFκB), negatively inotropic cytokines, like TNF and IL-1, are not synthesized. The postischemic contractile depression mediated by TNF and IL-1 is averted, and myofilament calcium sensitivity remains intact. Regardless of the mechanisms and signaling pathways involved in delayed preconditioning, the ultimate effect appears to be related to new protein synthesis that attenuates the inflammation associated with an ischemia-reperfusion injury, leading to reduced myocardial damage and subsequent improvement in myocardial function.

MYOCARDIAL STUNNING

Stunned myocardium is seen with a transient ischemic episode. The concept of "stunned" myocardium was first proposed in 1975 by Heyndrickx et al.[44] A brief ischemic insult results in depressed cardiac function that persists even after normalization of blood flow and resolution of electrocardiographic changes.[45] Stunning is typically found in areas adjacent to myocardial infarction and is often associated with angioplasty, cardiac surgery, coronary vasospasm, and unstable angina.[46] Stunned myocardium is characterized by hypocontractile myocardial segments with diminished functional reserve. Over time, stunned myocardium regains function. The duration of the ischemic insult determines the time and magnitude of recovery. Although thrombolytics, angioplasty, and coronary artery bypass grafting each reestablish healthy myocardial perfusion, reperfusion itself also provokes a destructive "oxidant burst" that may exacerbate the stunning within the affected myocardium.[28]

Multiple mediators and mechanisms have been implicated in myocardial stunning including abnormal calcium handling,[28] creation of oxygen-derived free radicals during reperfusion, prostacyclin, bradykinin, angiotensin-converting enzyme (ACE) activity, and local cytokine production.[47] Calcium levels are elevated soon after the onset of ischemia.[48] Intracellular ATP decreases, inhibiting sodium-calcium exchange, which further perturbs calcium homeostasis.[49] During early reperfusion, cytosolic calcium levels increase and exacerbate diastolic dysfunction by binding myocardial thin filaments and releasing intracellular proteases.[50] The secondary decrease in myocardial responsiveness to calcium and abnormal excitation-contraction coupling is associated with decreased intracellular calcium availability.[51] When calcium antagonists are given before an ischemic insult, stunning is attenuated.[52,53] The presence of increased cytosolic calcium and the formation of oxygen free radicals during myocardial reperfusion conspire to further delay recovery of the stunned myocardium.[54,55]

Even after the restoration of myocardial blood flow and normalization of the electrocardiogram, "stunned" myocardium continues to exhibit contractile dysfunction. Abnormal sarcoplasmic reticular function, decreased myofilament responsiveness to calcium, and protease release from neutrophils each contribute to stunning.[51] Abnormal contractile function is caused by a decreased availability of calcium from the sarcoplasmic reticulum and by a reduced responsiveness of the myofilaments to calcium as a result of troponin I proteolysis.[51] Although the level of cytosolic calcium

is likely normal in stunned myocardium, myofilament unrespon-
siveness to calcium is likely the cause of postischemic contractile
dysfunction.[56]

Multiple mechanisms lead to the formation of free radicals during reperfusion including xanthine oxidase, release of mitochondrial components, activated neutrophils, and production of
arachadonic acid metabolites.[57] We and others have reported that
antioxidants attenuate experimental myocardial stunning.[58,59]

The contribution of prostacyclin, bradykinin, and ACE activity to
myocardial stunning remains controversial. During acute ischemia
ACE activity increases, prompting vasoconstriction, bradykinin
breakdown, and prostacyclin production.[60] Prostacyclin is cardioprotective. Thus, there appears to be a balance between the cardio-
depressant effects of ACE and bradykinin and the protective effects
of prostacyclin. Administration of ACE inhibitors during or shortly
after an ischemic episode improves postischemic recovery.[61]

HIBERNATION

On restoration, by revascularization, of near-normal perfusion to a
chronically hypocontractile region, some zones recover function.
Myocardium capable of functional recovery with reperfusion is
termed hibernating. Recovery of contractile function may take several days or even weeks to months once blood flow is reestablished. This syndrome was first recognized when patients undergoing coronary artery bypass surgery who had preoperative left
ventricular dysfunction exhibited improvement in their left ventricular function after revascularization.[62,63] The mechanisms
responsible for hibernating myocardium have not been elucidated.
It was initially believed that a low-flow state created hibernating
myocardium. However, numerous studies have now confirmed
that hypoperfusion alone is not sufficient to account for hibernation. Additionally, hibernation most likely leads to a reduction in
blood flow as opposed to the reduction in flow leading to hibernation.[64-66] Chronic repeated ischemia or stunning may cause
myocardium to hibernate.[67,68]

Hibernation appears to be an adaptive response of the myocardium to ischemia. Hibernation involves the adaptive matching
of energy and oxygen consumption in an ischemic segment to the
available energy and oxygen supply.[69] For a portion of the myocardium to be hibernating, there must be chronically reduced coronary flow with associated (and perhaps compensatory) downregu-
lation of myocardial contractile function. The heart reaches a new
steady state relating perfusion (energy supply) to contraction

(energy demand), and the new steady state must be sufficient for cell viability.[70] This paradigm implies that the heart adapts to chronic hypoperfusion by reducing its energy requirements to match the energy supply, and the myocardium can achieve this new equilibrium before irreversible myocellular injury.

Metabolic changes rapidly occur to achieve the perfusion-contraction matching necessary for viable hibernation. Positron emission tomography (PET scanning) using ^{13}N ammonia and ^{15}O water confirms a decreased metabolic rate within hibernating myocardium. From the clinical standpoint, the discrimination between hibernating and irreversibly damaged myocardium is difficult but crucial.[71] The most widely used diagnostic tools are the thallium perfusion scan (indicates perfusion of viable cells), dobutamine echocardiography (exhibits inducible contractile function), electrocardiography (reflects only electrophysiologic status), and PET (confirms active myocellular metabolism). The PET scan using ^{13}NH$_3$ or H$_2$^{15}O is considered the "gold" standard in the diagnosis of hibernating myocardium and can predict the likelihood of muscle recovery after revascularization.[72]

Both functional and morphological changes occur within the myocardium after ischemia. An acute ischemic event initially provokes myofilament shortening and subsequent hypokinesis of the affected area. In addition, the feeding coronary arteries lose their ability to vasodilate in response to further ischemia. The arterial segments, which no longer can vasodilate, are typically distal to an area of stenosis. In hibernating myocardium, the number of sarcomeres in the affected area decreases. Ultrastructural changes also involve disorganization of the sarcoplasmic reticulum, loss of nuclear integrity, and overall dedifferentiation of the cell.[73-75] After revascularization, the time of recovery for hibernating myocardium ranges from minutes to months.[75]

MYOCARDIAL INFARCTION

With prolonged ischemia, the unprotected myocardium will sustain permanent damage. This irreversible necrosis or infarction has long-lasting effects on the global function and structure of the remaining viable myocardium. Sequelae that are seen with myocardial ischemia take time to develop, whereas other effects are seen immediately.

Apoptosis or "programmed cell death" in combination with necrosis appears to contribute to myocellular loss in ischemic heart disease.[76-78] After a myocardial infarction, the myocytes within the central portion of the ischemic zone undergo a necrotic death, whereas the myocytes surrounding the ischemic area exhibit apoptosis.[78] Apoptotic cardiomyocytes also reside within the central infarct zone and may account for as much as 33% of total myocyte loss.[79,80] Ischemia alone induces apoptosis, albeit to a lesser degree than ischemia followed by reperfusion.[81] Animal studies have demonstrated the upregulation of p53 transcription in rat ventricular myocytes.[82] p53 is a transcriptional activator protein that promotes DNA repair, but is also associated with apoptosis.[83]

The natural repair process after infarction is referred to as ventricular remodeling.[84] Remodeling is a myocardial strategy to compensate for the loss of contractile units. Some remodeling is adaptive and improves ventricular contractility, whereas some is maladaptive and can lead to further deterioration of cardiac function.

Left ventricular remodeling after an acute myocardial infarction can be both temporally and mechanistically divided into acute, subacute, and chronic.[84] The acute phase (within hours) consists of infarct zone wall thinning and chamber expansion. This phase is largely a structural result of the ischemia-reperfusion injury after the infarction. The subacute phase (several days) is characterized by an inflammatory reaction provoked by the necrotic myocytes. Scarring develops and the remaining viable myocytes begin to undergo hypertrophy. As the inflammatory reaction continues there is expansion of the infarct zone. As the scar tissue organizes there is further remodeling of the viable myocardium. This remodeling process promotes adjacent ventricular myocellular hypertrophy, which contributes to compensating for the loss of myocytes. This process can be adaptive in the case of small infarcts or may be maladaptive as with larger infarcts. When the infarction has caused the loss of a large number of contractile segments, the ventricle continues to dilate. With an increase in end-diastolic volume, a further augmentation in wall tension results in increased energy requirements for a decrease in ejection fraction. The role of apoptosis in ventricular remodeling is also prominent. Apoptotic myocytes have been identified in myocardium remote from the site of infarction. Human myocardium examined 10 days after an acute myocardial infarction contains apoptotic cardiomyocytes in areas of clearly unaffected myocardium.[85] The mediators responsible for inducing apoptosis within nonischemic myocardium are likely autocrine and paracrine cytokines such as endogenous TNF.[86] Apoptosis permits a clean cell death, which does not provoke infarction-expanding local inflammation.

Therapeutic interventions have been attempted to limit this deleterious postinfarction remodeling process. The majority have been aimed at reducing ventricular dilation by limiting the size of the infarct with early percutaneous transluminal angioplasty, coronary artery bypass grafting, or thrombolysis.[84] Medical therapy holds some promise in optimizing ventricular remodeling. ACE inhibitors are beneficial in reducing the risk of sudden death after an acute myocardial infarction.[87,88] The mechanism by which ACE inhibitors decrease mortality is related to the afterload reduction, which in effect limits infarct zone expansion and subsequent left ventricle dilation, remodeling, and hypertrophy.[89] In addition, patients taking ACE inhibitors have fewer postinfarction arrhythmias and electrocardiographic changes.

REFERENCES

1. Murry CE, Jennings RB, Reimer KA: Preconditioning with ischemia: A delay of lethal cell injury in ischemic myocardium. *Circulation* 74:1124-1136, 1986.
2. Kloner RA, Shook T, Przyklenk K, et al: Previous angina alters in-hospital outcome in TIMI 4: A clinical correlate to preconditioning [see comments]? *Circulation* 91:37-45, 1995.
3. Kerensky RA, Kutcher MA, Braden GA, et al: The effects of intra-coronary adenosine on preconditioning during coronary angioplasty. *Clin Cardiol* 18:91-96, 1995.
4. Tomai F, Crea F, Gaspardone A, et al: Mechanisms of cardiac pain during coronary angioplasty. *J Am Coll Cardiol* 22:1892-1896, 1993.
5. Kyriakidis MK, Petropoulakis PN, Tentolouris CA, et al: Relation between changes in blood flow of the contralateral coronary artery and the angiographic extent and function of recruitable collateral vessels arising from this artery during balloon coronary occlusion. *J Am Coll Cardiol* 23:869-878, 1994.
6. Deutsch E, Berger M, Kussmaul WG, et al: Adaptation to ischemia during percutaneous transluminal coronary angioplasty: Clinical, hemodynamic, and metabolic features [see comments]. *Circulation* 82:2044-2051, 1990.
7. Cribier A, Korsatz L, Koning R, et al: Improved myocardial ischemic response and enhanced collateral circulation with long repetitive coronary occlusion during angioplasty: A prospective study. *J Am Coll Cardiol* 20:578-586, 1992.
8. Alkhulaifi AM: Preconditioning the human heart. *Ann R Coll Surg Engl* 79:49-54, 1997.
9. Yellon DM, Baxter GF, Garcia-Dorado D, et al: Ischaemic preconditioning: Present position and future directions. *Cardiovasc Res* 37:21-33, 1998.
10. Marber MS, Latchman DS, Walker JM, et al: Cardiac stress protein elevation 24 hours after brief ischemia or heat stress is associated

with resistance to myocardial infarction. *Circulation* 88:1264-1272, 1993.

11. Meldrum DR, Cleveland JC Jr, Mitchell MB, et al: Protein kinase C mediates $Ca^{2(+)}$-induced cardioadaptation to ischemia-reperfusion injury. *Am J Physiol* 271:R718-R726, 1996.

12. Meldrum DR, Cleveland JC Jr, Meng X, et al: Protein kinase C isoform diversity in preconditioning. *J Surg Res* 69:183-187, 1997.

13. Meldrum DR, Cleveland JC Jr, Sheridan BC, et al: Differential effects of adenosine preconditioning on the postischemic rat myocardium. *J Surg Res* 65:159-164, 1996.

14. Rehring TF, Friese RS, Cleveland JC Jr, et al: Alpha-adrenergic preservation of myocardial pH during ischemia is PKC isoform dependent. *J Surg Res* 63:324-327, 1996.

15. Meldrum DR, Mitchell MB, Banerjee A, et al: Cardiac preconditioning: Induction of endogenous tolerance to ischemia-reperfusion injury. *Arch Surg* 128:1208-1211, 1993.

16. Banerjee A, Gamboni-Robertson F, Mitchell MB, et al: Stress-induced cardioadaptation reveals a code linking hormone receptors and spatial redistribution of PKC isoforms. *Ann N Y Acad Sci* 793:226-239, 1996.

17. Meng X, Brown JM, Ao L, et al: Norepinephrine induces cardiac heat shock protein 70 and delayed cardioprotection in the rat through alpha 1 adrenoceptors. *Cardiovasc Res* 32:374-383, 1996.

18. Cleveland JC Jr, Meldrum DR, Rowland RT, et al: Ischemic preconditioning of human myocardium: Protein kinase C mediates a permissive role for alpha 1-adrenoceptors. *Am J Physiol* 273:H902-H908, 1997.

19. Downey JM, Cohen MV: Signal transduction in ischemic preconditioning. *Z Kardiol* 84:77-86, 1995.

20. Gross GJ: ATP-sensitive potassium channels and myocardial preconditioning. *Basic Res Cardiol* 90:85-88, 1995.

21. Garlid KD, Paucek P, Yarov-Yarovoy V, et al: Cardioprotective effect of diazoxide and its interaction with mitochondrial ATP-sensitive K+ channels. Possible mechanism of cardioprotection. *Circ Res* 81:1072-1082, 1997.

22. Liu Y, Sato T, O'Rourke B, et al: Mitochondrial ATP-dependent potassium channels: Novel effectors of cardioprotection? *Circulation* 97:2463-2469, 1998.

23. Cleveland JC Jr, Meldrum DR, Cain BS, et al: Oral sulfonylurea hypoglycemic agents prevent ischemic preconditioning in human myocardium: Two paradoxes revisited. *Circulation* 96:29-32, 1997.

24. Grover GJ: Pharmacology of ATP-sensitive potassium channel (KATP) openers in models of myocardial ischemia and reperfusion. *Can J Physiol Pharmacol* 75:309-315, 1997.

25. Speechly-Dick ME, Grover GJ, Yellon DM: Does ischemic preconditioning in the human involve protein kinase C and the ATP-dependent K+ channel? Studies of contractile function after simu-

lated ischemia in an atrial in vitro model. *Circ Res* 77:1030-1035, 1995.

26. Cleveland JC Jr, Meldrum DR, Rowland RT, et al: Adenosine preconditioning of human myocardium is dependent upon the ATP-sensitive K+ channel. *J Mol Cell Cardiol* 29:175-182, 1997.
27. Cleveland JC Jr, Meldrum DR, Rowland RT, et al: The obligate role of protein kinase C in mediating clinically accessible cardiac preconditioning. *Surgery* 120:352-353, 1996.
28. Meldrum DR, Cleveland JC Jr, Sheridan BC, et al: Cardiac surgical implications of calcium dyshomeostasis in the heart. *Ann Thorac Surg* 61:1273-1280, 1996.
29. Miyawaki H, Ashraf M: Ca^{2+} as a mediator of ischemic preconditioning. *Circ Res* 80:790-799, 1997.
30. Meldrum DR, Cleveland JC Jr, Sheridan BC, et al: Cardiac preconditioning with calcium: Clinically accessible myocardial protection. *J Thorac Cardiovasc Surg* 112:778-786, 1996.
31. Meldrum DR: Mechanisms of cardiac preconditioning: Ten years after the discovery of ischemic preconditioning. *J Surg Res* 73:1-13, 1997.
32. Cleveland JC Jr, Wollmering MM, Meldrum DR, et al: Ischemic preconditioning in human and rat ventricle. *Am J Physiol* 271:H1786-H1794, 1996.
33. Cain BS, Meldrum DR, Meng X, et al: Therapeutic antidysrhythmic and functional protection in human atria. *J Surg Res* 76:143-148, 1998.
34. Cain BS, Meldrum DR, Meng X, et al: Calcium preconditioning in human myocardium. *Ann Thorac Surg* 65:1065-1070, 1998.
35. Banerjee A, Locke-Winter C, Rogers KB, et al: Preconditioning against myocardial dysfunction after ischemia and reperfusion by an alpha 1-adrenergic mechanism. *Circ Res* 73:656-670, 1993.
36. Mitchell MB, Meng X, Ao L, et al: Preconditioning of isolated rat heart is mediated by protein kinase C. *Circ Res* 76:73-81, 1995.
37. Miyawaki H, Zhou X, Ashraf M: Calcium preconditioning elicits strong protection against ischemic injury via protein kinase C signaling pathway. *Circ Res* 79:137-146, 1996.
38. Ashraf M, Suleiman J, Ahmad M: Ca^{2+} preconditioning elicits a unique protection against the Ca^{2+} paradox injury in rat heart: Role of adenosine. Fixed. *Circ Res* 74:360-367, 1994.
39. Cain BS, Meldrum DR, Harken AH: Protein kinase C in normal and pathologic myocardial states. *J Surg Res* 81:249-259, 1999.
40. Baxter GF, Goma FM, Yellon DM: Characterisation of the infarct-limiting effect of delayed preconditioning: Timecourse and dose-dependency studies in rabbit myocardium. *Basic Res Cardiol* 92:159-167, 1997.
41. Vegh A, Papp JG, Parratt JR: Prevention by dexamethasone of the marked antiarrhythmic effects of preconditioning induced 20 h after rapid cardiac pacing. *Br J Pharmacol* 113:1081-1082, 1994.

42. Tang XL, Qiu Y, Park SW, et al: Time course of late preconditioning against myocardial stunning in conscious pigs. *Circ Res* 79:424-434, 1996.

43. Baxter GF, Goma FM, Yellon DM: Involvement of protein kinase C in the delayed cytoprotection following sublethal ischaemia in rabbit myocardium. *Br J Pharmacol* 115:222-224, 1995.

44. Heyndrickx GR, Millard RW, McRitchie RJ, et al: Regional myocardial functional and electrophysiological alterations after brief coronary artery occlusion in conscious dogs. *J Clin Invest* 56:978-985, 1975.

45. Braunwald E, Kloner RA: The stunned myocardium: Prolonged, postischemic ventricular dysfunction. *Circulation* 66:1146-1149, 1982.

46. Hollenberg SM, Parrillo JE: Reversible causes of severe myocardial dysfunction. *J Heart Lung Transplant* 16:S7-S12, 1997.

47. Bolli R: Causative role of oxyradicals in myocardial stunning: A proven hypothesis. A brief review of the evidence demonstrating a major role of reactive oxygen species in several forms of postischemic dysfunction. *Basic Res Cardiol* 93:156-162, 1998.

48. Steenbergen C, Murphy E, Levy L, et al: Elevation in cytosolic free calcium concentration early in myocardial ischemia in perfused rat heart. *Circ Res* 60:700-707, 1987.

49. Du Toit J OL: Inhibitors of Ca^{++}-ATPase pump of sarcoplasmic reticulum attenuate reperfusion stunning in isolated rat heart. *J Cardiovasc Pharmacol* 24:678-684, 1994.

50. Atar D, Gao WD, Marban E: Alterations of excitation-contraction coupling in stunned myocardium and in failing myocardium. *J Mol Cell Cardiol* 27:783-791, 1995.

51. Marban E: Calcium homeostasis in stunned myocardium, in Heyndrick GR, Vatner SF, Wijns W (eds): *Stunning, Hibernation and Preconditioning.* Philadelphia, Lippincott-Raven, 1997, pp 195-204.

52. Opie L: Myocardial stunning: A role for calcium antagonists during reperfusion? *Cardiovasc Res* 26:20-24, 1992.

53. Opie LH: Should calcium antagonists be used after myocardial infarction? Ischemia selectivity versus vascular selectivity [see comments]. *Cardiovasc Drugs Ther* 6:19-24, 1992.

54. Xu KY, Zweier JL, Becker LC: Hydroxyl radical inhibits sarcoplasmic reticulum $Ca^{(2+)}$-ATPase function by direct attack on the ATP binding site. *Circ Res* 80:76-81, 1997.

55. Gao WD, Atar D, Liu Y, et al: Role of troponin I proteolysis in the pathogenesis of stunned myocardium. *Circ Res* 80:393-399, 1997.

56. Duncker DJ, Schulz R, Ferrari R, et al: "Myocardial stunning" remanining questions. *Cardiovasc Res* 38:549-558, 1998.

57. Bolli R: The early and late phases of preconditioning against myocardial stunning and the essential role of oxyradicals in the late phase: An overview. *Basic Res Cardiol* 91:57-63, 1996.

58. Bolli R: Oxygen-derived free radicals and myocardial reperfusion injury: An overview. *Cardiovasc Drugs Ther* 5:249S- 268S, 1991.

59. Brown JM, Terada LS, Grosso MA, et al: Xanthine oxidase produces hydrogen peroxide which contributes to reperfusion injury of

ischemic, isolated, perfused rat hearts. *J Clin Invest* 81:1297-1301, 1988.

60. Ertl G, Alexander RW, Kloner RA: Interactions between coronary occlusion and the renin-angiotensin system in the dog. *Basic Res Cardiol* 78:518-533, 1983.

61. Przyklenk K, Kloner RA: "Cardioprotection" by ACE-inhibitors in acute myocardial ischemia and infarction? *Basic Res Cardiol* 88:139-154, 1993.

62. Rahimtoola SH: Coronary bypass surgery for chronic angina: 1981. A perspective. *Circulation* 65:225-241, 1982.

63. Rahimtoola SH: A perspective on the three large multicenter randomized clinical trials of coronary bypass surgery for chronic stable angina. *Circulation* 72:V123-V135, 1985.

64. Mills I, Fallon JT, Wrenn D, et al: Adaptive responses of coronary circulation and myocardium to chronic reduction in perfusion pressure and flow. *Am J Physiol* 266:H447-H457, 1994.

65. Berman M, Fischman AJ, Southern J, et al: Myocardial adaptation during and after sustained, demand-induced ischemia: Observations in closed-chest, domestic swine. *Circulation* 94:755-762, 1996.

66. Vanoverschelde JL, Wijns W, Borgers M, et al: Chronic myocardial hibernation in humans: From bedside to bench. *Circulation* 95:1961-1971, 1997.

67. Shen YT, Vatner SF: Mechanism of impaired myocardial function during progressive coronary stenosis in conscious pigs: Hibernation versus stunning? *Circ Res* 76:479-488, 1995.

68. Vanoverschelde JL, Wijns W, Depre C, et al: Mechanisms of chronic regional postischemic dysfunction in humans: New insights from the study of noninfarcted collateral-dependent myocardium [see comments]. *Circulation* 87:1513-1523, 1993.

69. Heusch G, Schulz R: Hibernating myocardium: A review. *J Mol Cell Cardiol* 28:2359-2372, 1996.

70. Rahimtoola SH: The hibernating myocardium [see comments]. *Am Heart J* 117:211-221, 1989.

71. Vanoverschelde JL, Melin JA, Bol A, et al: Regional oxidative metabolism in patients after recovery from reperfused anterior myocardial infarction: Relation to regional blood flow and glucose uptake. *Circulation* 85:9-21, 1992.

72. Niroomand F, Kubler W: Hibernating, stunning and ischemic preconditioning of the myocardium: Therapeutic implications. *Clin Invest* 72:731-736, 1994.

73. Ausma J, Furst D, Thone F, et al: Molecular changes of titin in left ventricular dysfunction as a result of chronic hibernation. *J Mol Cell Cardiol* 27:1203-1212, 1995.

74. Ausma J, Cleutjens J, Thone F, et al: Chronic hibernating myocardium: Interstitial changes. *Mol Cell Biochem* 147:35-42, 1995.

75. Camici PG, Wijns W, Borgers M, et al: Pathophysiological mechanisms of chronic reversible left ventricular dysfunction due to coro-

nary artery disease (hibernating myocardium). *Circulation* 96:3205-3214, 1997.

76. Itoh G, Tamura J, Suzuki M, et al: DNA fragmentation of human infarcted myocardial cells demonstrated by the nick end labeling method and DNA agarose gel electrophoresis. *Am J Pathol* 146:1325-1331, 1995.

77. Bardales RH, Hailey LS, Xie SS, et al: In situ apoptosis assay for the detection of early acute myocardial infarction. *Am J Pathol* 149:821-829, 1996.

78. Saraste A, Pulkki K, Kallajoki M, et al: Apoptosis in human acute myocardial infarction. *Circulation* 95:320-323, 1997.

79. Fliss H, Gattinger D: Apoptosis in ischemic and reperfused rat myocardium. *Circ Res* 79:949-956, 1996.

80. Bialik S, Geenen DL, Sasson IE, et al: Myocyte apoptosis during acute myocardial infarction in the mouse localizes to hypoxic regions but occurs independently of p53. *J Clin Invest* 100:1363-1372, 1997.

81. Tanaka M, Ito H, Adachi S, et al: Hypoxia induces apoptosis with enhanced expression of Fas antigen messenger RNA in cultured neonatal rat cardiomyocytes. *Circ Res* 75:426-433, 1994.

82. Long X, Boluyt MO, Hipolito ML, et al: p53 and the hypoxia-induced apoptosis of cultured neonatal rat cardiac myocytes. *J Clin Invest* 99:2635-2643, 1997.

83. Haunstetter A, Izumo S: Apoptosis: Basic mechanisms and implications for cardiovascular disease. *Circ Res* 82:1111-1129, 1998.

84. Maisch B: Ventricular remodeling. *Cardiology* 87:2-10, 1996.

85. Olivetti G, Quaini F, Sala R, et al: Acute myocardial infarction in humans is associated with activation of programmed myocyte cell death in the surviving portion of the heart. *J Mol Cell Cardiol* 28:2005-2016, 1996.

86. Meldrum DR: Tumor necrosis factor in the heart. *Am J Physiol* 274:R577-R595, 1998.

87. Pfeffer MA, Braunwald E, Moye LA, et al: Effect of captopril on mortality and morbidity in patients with left ventricular dysfunction after myocardial infarction: Results of the survival and ventricular enlargement trial. The SAVE Investigators [see comments]. *N Engl J Med* 327:669-677, 1992.

88. Latini R, Maggioni AP, Zuanetti G: Myocardial infarction: When and how should we initiate treatment with ACE inhibitors? GISSI-3 Investigators. *Cardiology* 87:16-22, 1996.

89. Bassand JP: Left ventricular remodelling after acute myocardial infarction: Solved and unsolved issues. *Eur Heart J* 16:58-63, 1995.

CHAPTER 3

Robotically Assisted Endoscopic Coronary Artery Bypass Grafting: Current State of the Art

Ralph J. Damiano, Jr, MD
Professor and Chief, Department of Cardiothoracic Surgery,
Pennsylvania State University; Chief, Section of Cardiothoracic Surgery,
Penn State Geisinger Health System, Hershey, Pennsylvania

Hermann Reichenspurner, MD, PhD
Associate Professor, Department of Cardiothoracic Surgery, Ludwig-
Maximilians Universitat, Klinikum Grosshadern, Munich, Germany

Christopher T. Ducko, MD
Senior Resident, Surgery, Pennsylvania State University; Penn State
Geisinger Health System, Hershey, Pennsylvania

The introduction and widespread acceptance of minimally invasive techniques have revolutionized many surgical disciplines during the last two decades. Endoscopic operations have been shown to reduce patient morbidity and provide a more rapid recovery. Until recently, these endoscopic approaches have had little impact on the field of cardiac surgery. However, during the past few years, less invasive cardiac procedures that eliminate the median sternotomy or cardiopulmonary bypass have been introduced and are rapidly gaining acceptance.[1,2] Unfortunately, the ultimate minimally invasive procedure (ie, totally endoscopic closed-chest coronary artery bypass grafting) has not been possible because of several shortcomings associated with conventional endoscopic surgery. These include limited access to and visualization of target vessels, absence of force feedback, the length and imprecision of endoscopic instruments, and the magnification of cardiac motion. Currently available robotic systems and computer assistance represent an enabling technology that has the potential to allow surgeons to perform endoscopic coronary artery bypass grafting (ECABG). This chapter will summarize the present state of the art of this rapidly growing field.

ROBOTIC SURGICAL SYSTEMS

Robotic systems have been developed to assist in endoscopic suturing. These systems consist of three main components: a sur-

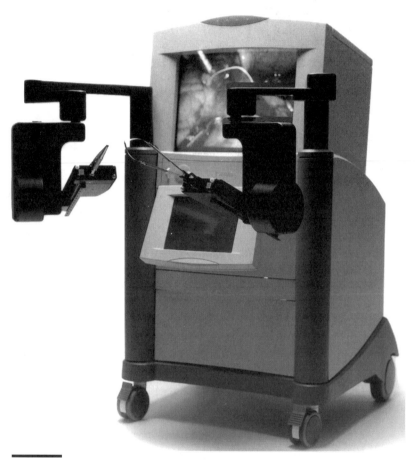

FIGURE 1.
The ZEUS Robotic Surgical System Surgeon Interface Device (Computer Motion, Inc, Goleta, Calif). This consists of a video monitor and two instrument handles that can be customized. The surgeon manipulates the instrument handles. A computer controller digitizes the surgeon's motions and relays this information in real-time to robotic arms.

geon interface device, a computer controller, and specially designed instrument tips attached to robotic arms (Figs 1 and 2). The surgeon manipulates traditional surgical instrument handles from the interface device. His movements are relayed to a computer controller that digitizes these motions and relays this information in real-time to computer-driven robotic arms which are attached to the operating room table. These robotic arms hold specially designed endoscopic instruments that are placed through small ports (5-10 mm). These computer-guided systems can control both surgical instruments and endoscopic cameras.

The principal difference between robotically assisted and traditional surgery is that a computer is integrated between the instrument handle and instrument tip. The computer digitizes the surgeon's movements and is able to perfect the digital signal with fil-

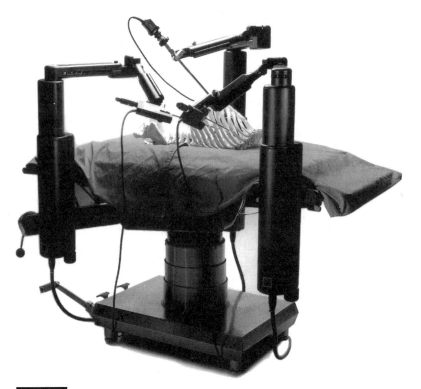

FIGURE 2.

The robotic arms are attached to the operating room table and precisely control instrument tips that are positioned via ports within the surgical field. Two arms hold the surgical instruments, and a third arm is used to control the endoscope.

tering and motion scaling. The surgeon also visualizes the operative field with an endoscope, and views the image on a video monitor. There are several advantages that are inherent to this new digital operative environment.

ADVANTAGES OF ROBOTIC ASSISTANCE
MAGNIFICATION AND IMPROVED VISUALIZATION

Most conventional cardiac procedures are performed with the assistance of surgical loupes. The magnification typically available with these glasses is 2.5× to 3.0×. With standard endoscope and camera configurations, a much greater magnification (10×-20×) can be achieved. This extra magnification can enhance visualization and anatomical detail, especially when working on small vessels. A drawback of endoscopy for microsurgical applications has been the loss of depth perception with 2-dimensional video monitors.[3] However, several companies now offer high-resolution 3-dimensional video systems for endoscopic surgical applications (Fig 3). These cameras are able to be introduced through ports (<10 mm) and allow for excellent visualization during endoscopic microsurgery.[4-7]

Another technological advancement in endoscopic visualization has been the development of a robotic arm (AESOP, Computer Motion, Inc, Goleta, Calif) that is capable of manipulating the endoscope.[8] With this system, the surgeon benefits both from endoscopic visualization and voice-activated camera control, thus eliminating the need for an assistant. Kavoussi et al[9] have shown that the robotic camera arm can more effectively manipulate and control the video endoscope than a human assistant during laparoscopic procedures. Additionally, Geis et al[10] found that requirements for camera lens cleaning during procedures are reduced by three- to fivefold when a robotic arm is used. Not only is this system more stable and precise than manually guided videoscopic assistance, but its movements can be voice controlled by the surgeon, and ideal camera positions can be saved and returned to with a simple command. This technology is already in use in minimally invasive cardiac surgical procedures.[11,12]

IMPROVED DEXTERITY

Involuntary tremor can be a significant hindrance when performing cardiac surgical procedures, especially when working in a magnified field with long endoscopic instruments. The robotic systems currently in use today are capable of eliminating this problem. By using a computer controller to digitize surgical movement, high-frequency motion can be filtered, allowing the sur-

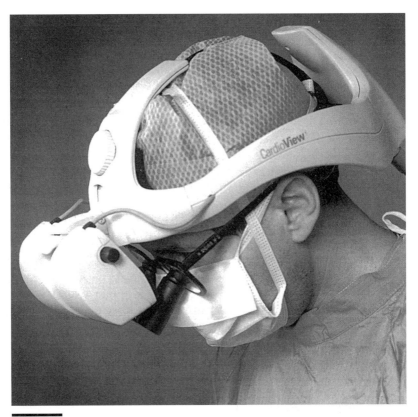

FIGURE 3.
The head-mounted display developed by Vista Medical Technologies (Westborough, Mass) that integrates 3-dimensional visualization of surgical anatomy and related diagnostic and monitoring data. (Courtesy of Vista Medical Technologies.)

geon's motions to be translated into smooth movements free of tremor.

Another advantage of robotically assisted cardiac surgery lies in the ability of the computer interface to scale the surgeon's movements. This allows for gross hand movements at the console to be translated into fine movements by the robotic instruments at the operative site. The computer controllers used in many robotic systems permit a variable degree of motion scaling (from 1:1 to 10:1), depending on surgeon preference. As magnification increases, scaling can be increased allowing the surgeon to feel that he is being shrunk down into the operative field. This is called "scaled telepresence" and enables surgeons to operate comfortably on extremely small structures.

IMPROVED INSTRUMENTATION

Computer-assisted instrumentation has advantages over conventional hand-held instruments. Movement of hand-held instruments is often limited by the way in which the instruments become fulcrums, working around pivot points based on trocar positioning. By separating the instrument tip from the handle, this phenomenon is eliminated. Traditional endoscopic instruments require the surgeon to move the handle in the reverse direction that the instrument tip is intended to travel. Robotic systems automatically rectify this and allow for intuitive hand movements in which the instrument tip follows the movement of the handle at the surgeon console.

Some systems also offer two more degrees of freedom than conventional instruments by including a "wrist" joint to facilitate more natural handlike articulation. This design is comparable to the human hand-arm system and allows for the wristlike motions made by the surgeon at the console to be reproduced at the tip of the instrument.[13] The Intuitive Surgical telemanipulation system (Intuitive Surgical, Mountain View, Calif), which operates with six degrees of freedom, is one such example (Fig 4). An additional advanced feature of some robotic systems is the ability to provide the surgeon with haptic feedback.[14] This sense of touch is helpful to achieve a realistic interface between the surgeon and the operative field.

IMPROVED ERGONOMICS

In conventional endoscopic surgery, many factors contribute to operator fatigue. From a physical standpoint, the surgeon is required to stand at the operating table, often in awkward positions, based on trocar placement. The video monitor is across the table and may not be positioned conveniently for direct, unobstructed viewing. As a result, surgeons often complain of back and neck stiffness, and performance may suffer.

In robotically assisted surgery, many of these drawbacks are avoided because the surgeon is seated directly in front of a console. Regardless of the video display format (2- or 3-dimensional visualization, video monitor or head-mounted system), the monitor device is directly in front of the surgeon. This interface style immerses the surgeon in the operative field without intrusions or distractions, thereby providing the surgeon the ability for greater focus and concentration. Additionally, the surgeon operates while seated, in a chair ergonomically designed for the reduction of physical fatigue. With less fatigue, the surgeon's performance should remain optimal for longer periods of time.

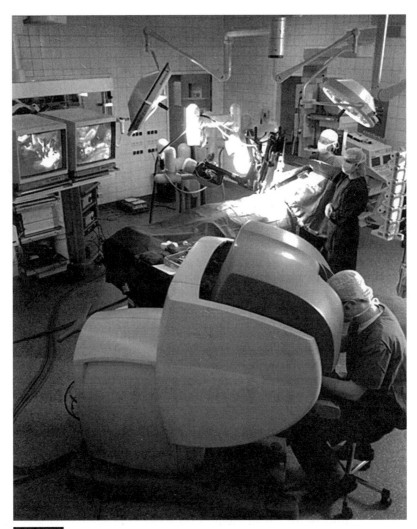

FIGURE 4.
A picture of the Intuitive Surgical DaVinci System (Intuitive Surgical, Mountain View, Calif) installed at University of Leipzig. (Courtesy of Intuitive Surgical.)

ENHANCED PRECISION

With better visualization, improved dexterity, and reduced fatigue, robotically assisted cardiac surgery should allow for a level of precision superior to that attainable with conventional endoscopic instrumentation. This may allow endoscopic techniques to be applied for the first time to microsurgical, reconstructive surgical specialties. Preliminary work has shown that precise anastomoses are possible when the advantages of robotic surgery are applied to totally ECABG.[7,15,16]

EXPERIMENTAL RESULTS

The two systems currently at the forefront of robotic cardiac surgery are the DaVinci telemanipulation system from Intuitive Surgical (Fig 4) and the ZEUS Robotic Surgical System developed by Computer Motion, Inc (Figs 1 and 2). Each system enables the surgeon to manipulate instruments in real-time on a remote operative field, to which he is linked only by a computer system.[17] Preliminary inanimate, ex vivo, and in vivo studies have documented the efficacy of these systems.

INANIMATE STUDIES

Garcia-Ruiz et al[18] used a custom-made plastic heart model to evaluate performance enhancement using the ZEUS system in creating a coronary artery bypass anastomosis. Two tubular polyurethane structures (3-mm diameter) were used to simulate an end-to-side anastomosis. All anastomoses were patent and without obstruction. Falk et al[19] recently completed a study using the Intuitive Surgical telemanipulation system. They hypothesized that general positioning and orientation in space would be attained more effectively with six degrees of freedom compared with four. In an endoscopic trainer model, both time and error rates were significantly less using a robotic system with six degrees of freedom.

EX VIVO STUDIES

Using a prototype telepresence surgery system developed by Green et al[20] at the Stanford Research Institute, Bowersox et al[21] performed feasibility studies in animals to investigate vascular applications of this technology. This work consisted of ex vivo studies in which the robotic system was used to close 3-cm arteriotomies in excised bovine aortas, and also included intact animal studies in which the surgeon isolated the porcine common femoral artery and performed and closed a 2-cm arteriotomy.

Although the times required for arteriotomy closure with this prototype telepresence surgery system were more than double that using conventional techniques, further studies showed that force feedback and stereoscopic video display were important for achieving intuitive performance with the telesurgery system.[22] These early studies showed that vascular surgery performed by a remotely located surgeon was feasible.

This initial prototype system evolved into a more advanced telemanipulation system currently available from Intuitive Surgical. Early feasibility work using this system has been done by Shennib et al,[23] who tested this telemanipulation technology in an ex vivo porcine heart model. The circumflex coronary artery was dissected and grafted to the left anterior descending coronary artery (LAD) using the Intuitive system. The anastomoses (n = 6) were performed in 14.6 ± 2.6 minutes, and all were fully patent.

Stephenson et al[24] used an early prototype of the ZEUS system to perform anastomoses between the dissected right coronary artery and the in situ LAD in excised pig hearts (n = 25). All anastomoses were successfully performed and found to be patent with precise suture placement. This preliminary cadaver work in a custom-made thoracic simulator was used to determine appropriate thoracoscopic port placement and orientation before embarking on in vivo animal studies.

In an effort to document the advantages of robotically assisted surgery, Shennib et al[7] recently performed anastomoses in the ex vivo porcine heart model using five different techniques. Four of the techniques involved the use of conventional or endoscopic instruments with either direct vision using surgical loupes, or indirect vision using a head-mounted 3-dimensional video system (Vista Medical Technologies, Westborough, Mass); the fifth technique involved the use of the Intuitive Surgical robotic system.

The times for anastomosis using endoscopic instruments with either direct vision or the 3-dimensional system were 21.1 ± 2.1 and 22.4 ± 3.0 minutes, respectively. Using conventional instruments with surgical loupes or the 3-dimensional headset resulted in significantly faster anastomotic times of 6.7 ± 0.5 and 10.5 ± 1.6 minutes, respectively. The time for performance of the anastomosis with the Intuitive Surgical system was 8.9 ± 1.4 minutes. Although sewing under direct vision with conventional instruments was performed significantly faster than in all other groups ($P < .04$), robotically assisted anastomotic times were comparable to the group using the 3-dimensional system with conventional instruments.

Falk et al[16] also used the Intuitive Surgical robotic system to test the efficacy of performing robotically assisted coronary anastomoses. In a randomized double-blind study on excised pig hearts, this computer-assisted technology was compared with conventional manually performed anastomoses. The mean time for completion of anastomoses was 12 minutes using the robotic system, with a 100% patency rate.

IN VIVO STUDIES

An acute animal study was performed using a bovine cardiopulmonary bypass model to examine the efficacy of ECABG using the ZEUS system.[25] A small 3-cm left subcostal incision was made, and the left internal thoracic artery was harvested endoscopically. Three access ports were used to sew the anastomosis (Fig 5). A 10-mm camera was placed through a right paramedian subxiphoid port, while the two 5-mm instruments were placed through subcostal ports, 7 cm on either side of the camera port (the small, left subcostal incision was closed before port placement). A continuous end-to-side anastomosis between the left internal thoracic artery and LAD was performed using the robotic system (Fig 6). The animals (n = 8) were weaned from bypass, and flow measurements were obtained before they were killed. Excised hearts and grafts were submitted for angiographic and pathologic evaluations. The mean anastomotic time was 33.9 ± 1.9 minutes. All anastomoses were patent by angiography, and microscopic evaluation revealed no thrombi or other abnormalities.

The favorable results of this study led us to perform a long-term study following a similar protocol to assess graft patency.[15]

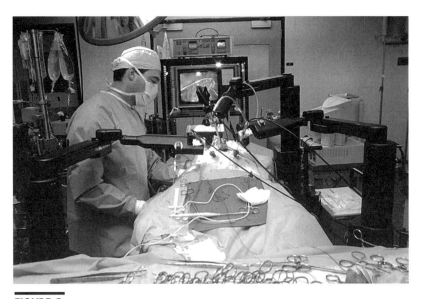

FIGURE 5.
The ZEUS Microsurgical Robotic System in position during an acute bovine case. The robotic arm holding the camera is in the middle; the two arms holding the surgical instruments are on each side. All three ports are placed subcostally. (Courtesy of Computer Motion, Inc, Goleta, Calif.)

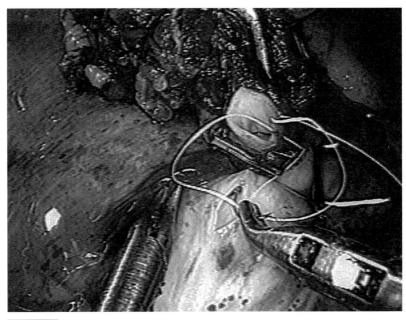

FIGURE 6.
Intraoperative photograph taken from the endoscopic camera of the left internal mammary artery to left anterior descending anastomosis in a calf.

Surviving animals (n = 6) recovered without complications and underwent necropsy at 31 ± 2 days postoperatively. Chronic angiographic graft patency was 100%, with a graft flow of 38.5 ± 5.0 mL/min. This study validated the feasibility of robotically assisted ECABG in a clinically relevant model, demonstrating excellent short-term graft patency.

As a result of the promising experimental results, clinical trials with robotic technology are currently underway and are summarized in the next sections.

INITIAL US CLINICAL EXPERIENCE

The Food and Drug Administration approved a prospective single-center clinical trial at Penn State University to evaluate the efficacy and safety of robotically assisted ECABG. Permission was granted to study 10 patients undergoing robotically assisted endoscopic anastomosis of the left internal mammary artery (LIMA) to the LAD. Primary outcome measurements were device-related complications and graft patency at 6 to 8 weeks. After approval from our institutional review board, a total of 15 patients were enrolled in

TABLE 1.
Exclusion Criteria

1. Patients older than 80 years.
2. Patients with an ejection fraction of 40% or less.
3. Severe noncardiac conditions.
4. Severe peripheral vascular disease.
5. Myocardial infarction within 7 days before procedure.
6. Patients undergoing concomitant surgery, emergency surgery, or who have had previous thoracic surgery.
7. Calcified or diffuse disease in the left anterior descending coronary artery.
8. Patients participating in other investigational device or drug studies.

the trial. Patients were considered eligible if they (1) had angiographic evidence of occlusive disease of the LAD; (2) required elective or urgent CABG surgery; and (3) had not undergone previous cardiac surgery. Five enrolled patients were excluded from participation by criteria listed in Table 1.

Nine of the 10 patients underwent standard median sternotomy and the LIMA was taken down in the traditional manner. These patients required other bypass grafts, which were done using standard open techniques. In the tenth patient, the LIMA was harvested thoracoscopically through three endoscopic ports. A small anterior thoracotomy was then made in the third intercostal space, and the patient underwent bypass using the Heartport System (Redwood City, Calif). All patients underwent endoscopic surgery using the ZEUS Robotic Microsurgical System. Three ports were inserted to perform the anastomosis (Fig 7). A 5-mm right instrument port was placed in the midline just below the xiphoid process. A 10-mm camera port was placed approximately 7 cm lateral to the midline port in the fifth or sixth intercostal space. The 5-mm left instrument port was placed 7 cm lateral to the camera port in the sixth or seventh intercostal space along the anterior axillary line. A 0-degree endoscope was used and was attached to the AESOP voice-controlled robotic arm.

In those patients who required grafts in addition to the LIMA to LAD anastomosis, these grafts were performed first using traditional open-chest methods. After this, the heart was left in situ, and the chest retractor was relaxed to allow a more anatomical position of the chest wall. An arteriotomy was made in the distal LAD using specialized endoscopic scissors. A continuous end-to-side anastomosis was performed endoscopically using the robotic instruments (Fig 8). No manipulation of the heart was necessary to perform the anastomosis, and there was excellent visualization of each stitch through the subxiphoid camera port. A running anastomosis was performed with specially designed 7-cm, double-armed, 7-0 Gore-Tex suture (WL Gore & Assoc, Flagstaff, Ariz). On completion of the anastomosis, the patients were weaned from bypass. Blood flow was measured in the graft using an ultrasonic flow probe and flow meter (HT311, Transonic Systems, Inc, Ithaca, NY). If flow was not judged to be adequate, selective angiography was performed in the operating room suite.

Of the 10 patients, there were 6 men and 4 women. The average age was 55.8 ± 3 years. Their ejection fraction averaged 50% ± 4%. The robotic system was quick and easy to assemble. The average time required for setup was 14.9 ± 2.1 minutes. There were no

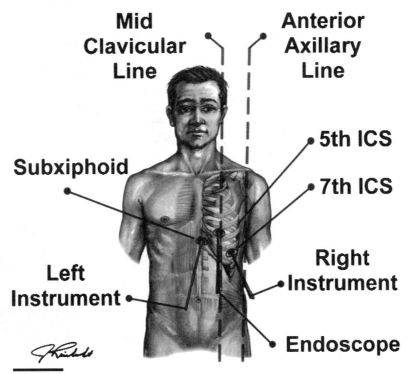

FIGURE 7.
Port placement in the 10 patients undergoing endoscopic coronary artery bypass grafting at Penn State University. *Abbreviation: ICS,* Intercostal space.

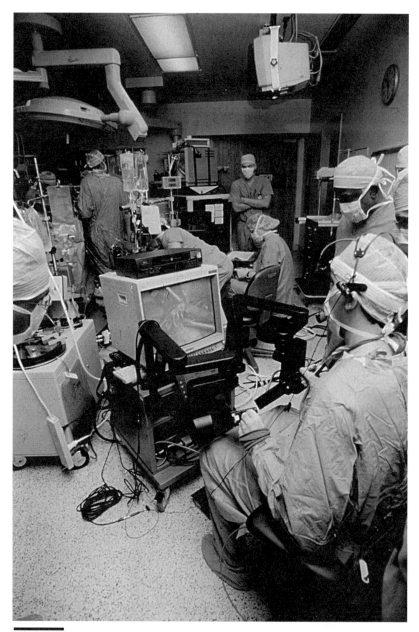

FIGURE 8.
Intraoperative photograph of the surgeon performing robotically assisted
endoscopic cardiac surgery. The surgeon is seated at an interface device
that is approximately 5 yards from the patient. The operating room table
can be seen in the background.

intraoperative complications related to port placement. There were no mechanical failures of the robotic system.

The total number of grafts performed was 2.3 ± 0.3 per patient with a mean cross-clamp time of 51.1 ± 1.6 minutes. The time required to perform the endoscopic LIMA to LAD anastomosis of the robotic system was 23.6 ± 1.4 minutes (range, 18-30 minutes). All anastomoses were successfully performed and no repair stitches were required. Eighty percent of the grafts measured were patent and had excellent diastolic flow by ultrasound. Average graft flow was 31 ± 7 mL/min. Two of the grafts had inadequate flow and were taken down and reconstructed manually. In one case, an intraoperative angiogram was performed and the graft was not visualized. However, the distal anastomosis was probe patent. In the second case, angiography was unavailable. Subsequent review of the videotape revealed a technical error.

There was only one postoperative complication. This patient required return to the operating room on the evening of surgery for excessive mediastinal hemorrhage. No other complications were encountered in the postoperative period. The average length of stay in the ICU was 1.1 ± 1 days. The average length of stay in the hospital was 4.1 ± 0.2 days.

There has been 100% late follow-up. The mean period of follow-up was 182 ± 10.7 days. There have been no late complications, and all patients are presently New York Heart Association Class I. Eight weeks after surgery, graft patency was assessed by repeat coronary angiography. These studies were all performed at our institution and showed that 100% of the LIMA to LAD grafts were patent (Fig 9).

This trial has demonstrated the feasibility of ECABG. There were no device-related complications, and coronary anastomoses can be performed with robotic assistance with acceptable short-term results.

EARLY EUROPEAN EXPERIENCE WITH ROBOTIC TECHNOLOGY

Computer and robotically assisted coronary artery surgery was started in Europe in April 1998. At the University Hospitals in Broussais and Leipzig, the Intuitive Surgical robotic system was used for mitral and coronary artery surgery. The first closed-chest CABG was done at the Hospital Broussais a few weeks later.[26] At the University of Leipzig, a total of 40 procedures using the Intuitive Surgical robotic system were reported in 1999 at the Annual Meeting of the International Society for Minimally Invasive Cardiac Surgery in Paris.[27] Of 40 robotically assisted

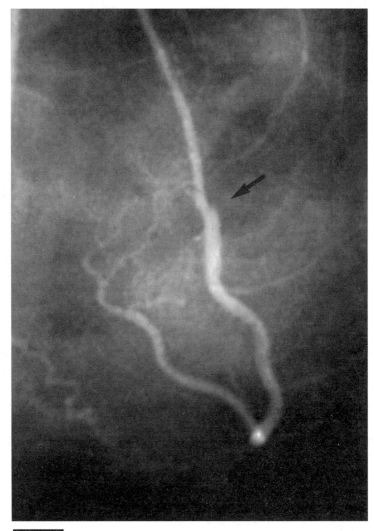

FIGURE 9.
Angiogram at 8 weeks of a robotically sewn left internal mammary artery to left anterior descending graft. The anastomotic site is marked by the *arrow*.

CABG procedures, 9 were done completely endoscopically using three small incisions (2 cm per incision). At the University of Dresden, a second group has recently started performing both open- and closed-chest CABG using the Intuitive Surgical system. Up to June 1999, a total of 30 surgeries were performed including 6 closed-chest procedures.[28]

At the University of Munich, the ZEUS system has been used since July 1998.[29] After initial cadaveric and animal studies, 18 patients were evaluated for robotically assisted CABG anastomosis. Five of these patients underwent an endoscopic approach. In these cases, harvesting of the LIMA was performed endoscopically. Two patients were placed on Port-Access (Heartport, Redwood City, Calif) cardiopulmonary bypass. The other 3 patients had beating heart surgery using endoscopic stabilizers. The remaining 12 patients were operated on through a sternotomy with (n = 9) or without (n = 3) the use of cardiopulmonary bypass (Octopus, Medtronic, Inc, Minneapolis, Minn) using a suction stabilizer. In all cases, the bypass grafts (LIMA to LAD in all cases, additional vein grafts to the diagonal branch in 4 cases, and to the obtuse marginal branch in 2 cases) were anastomosed endoscopically with the ZEUS system through three thoracic ports.

In the clinical series, one case was switched to a manual anastomosis because of a small LAD. In the endoscopic cases, LIMA preparation times ranged from 69 to 110 minutes (mean, 82 minutes). In all cases, the total operating room time ranged from 4 to 7 hours (median, 4.5 hours). The times for the endoscopic coronary artery anastomosis ranged from 14 to 42 minutes (mean, 21 minutes), with no difference between the arrested heart versus the beating heart procedures. Postoperative length of stay ranged from 4 to 20 days (median, 6.0 days), and stay in the ICU ranged from 0.5 to 15 days (median, 1.0 days). Postoperative complications included one case of reversible postoperative delirium and a case of adult respiratory distress syndrome, requiring prolonged ventilation. All patients had uneventful postoperative angiography 4 days to 6 weeks after surgery and were discharged in excellent condition.

Although dramatic progress has been made in the development of ECABG during the last 2 years, we are still a long way from its widespread applicability in cardiac surgery. Many challenges lie ahead of us to make this a reproducible, commonly performed operation. Particularly, we need to find a way to judge preoperatively whether a patient is an appropriate candidate and, if so, what is the correct port placement. We must improve and simplify the operative choreography of endoscopic procedures to shorten the operating time. We must develop techniques and access vessels other than the LAD, because most patients have multivessel disease. To be truly minimally invasive, we also must learn to perform these procedures on the beating heart. This will be a challenge considering the limited space inside the thorax. Finally, we must strive to make ECABG cost-effective and affordable. This will require a close partnership between surgeons and industry. All of these goals are achievable; however, they will require hard work and innovation on the part of cardiac surgeons, engineers, and industry to make the dream of ECABG a reality for the majority of our patients.

FUTURE DIRECTIONS

The real significance of robotically assisted cardiac surgery lies in the resultant integration of computers into our operating rooms. Our specialty will be fundamentally changed by this phenomenon. Gordon Moore, the cofounder of Intel Corporation, predicted in the early 1970s that computer processing power would double every 18 months. In fact, the computer industry has exceeded this goal, and this has led to dramatic changes throughout our society. What are the implications of Moore's Law as we enter into an era of computer-assisted and computer-guided surgery? The principal result will be rapid change and startling advances in surgeon control, imaging capability, and information access.

The improvements in surgeon control with computer-assisted surgery will be dramatic. Robotic and computer assistance have the potential to enhance surgical ability and allow cardiothoracic surgeons not only to perform present procedures better, but to perform procedures that heretofore have been impossible because of our inherent technical shortcomings. Robotically assisted cardiac surgery is a good example of the power of this technology. Despite many efforts during the last 10 years, endoscopic coronary surgery has not been possible with traditional, hand-held instruments. With computer-assisted tremor elimination and motion scaling, we are now able to reproducibly perform this procedure.

These improvements in surgeon control will be coupled directly with equally important improvements in imaging capability in the operating room, allowing for both the planning and performance of surgical procedures. In thoracic surgery, this may include 3-dimensional echocardiography, spiral CT scans, angiography, fluoroscopy, and MRI. As we no longer will work through large incisions, we will use these images to help guide our procedures. In the future, advanced video interfaces will allow for manipulation of the image to benefit the surgeon and facilitate the procedure.[30] With sophisticated image fusion technology, it may be possible to view the echocardiogram, angiogram, or CT scan directly on the video monitor and, if needed, superimpose these on the visual field. These images fused with our endoscopic pictures may allow surgeons to precisely define intracardiac and extracardiac anatomy without the need for direct visualization. In this type of environment, cardiothoracic surgeons may find themselves working closely with our medical colleagues as intravascular and extravascular interventions may be carried on simultaneously on the same patient.

Because we will have a digital visual interface between us and the patient, it may also be possible to operate on a beating heart while working in "virtual stillness." By gating the movement of the robotic camera and arms to the heartbeat, the motion could be effectively canceled, increasing surgical precision.

Finally, and most importantly, there will be improvements in information access. In the operating room, this will consist of networked video monitors that provide access to the hospital information system and ancillary services (ie, radiology, cardiac catheterization laboratory, echocardiography), as well as to local area networks, the Internet, and the hospital library. This technology will also allow for experts to assist their colleagues throughout the world, via high-speed video links. This has the potential to decrease patient morbidity and shorten recovery times. Moreover, these new approaches will allow our specialty to remain competitive with improving alternative therapies (ie, angioplasty, gene therapy).

As surgeons, our challenge will be to not be pigeonholed as technicians who work through incisions, but instead to see ourselves as cardiothoracic interventionalists who are able to perform percutaneous interventions on various intrathoracic structures. We may play a key role in the future in gene therapy, angiogenesis, arrhythmia ablation, and other areas not traditionally thought of as the domain of the surgeon. The era of computer-assisted surgery has begun and promises to be one of startling advances in our capability as cardiac surgeons. Robotics and computer assistance have the potential to transform both our operating rooms and our specialty as we enter the new millenium.

REFERENCES

1. Subramanian VA, McMabe JC, Geller CM: Minimally invasive direct coronary artery bypass grafting: Two-year clinical experience. *Ann Thorac Surg* 64:1648-1655, 1997.
2. Calafiore AM, DiGiammarco G, Teodori G, et al: Recent advances in multivessel coronary grafting without cardiopulmonary bypass. *Heart Surgery Forum* 1:20-25, 1998.
3. Peitgen K, Walz MV, Walz MV, et al: A prospective randomized experimental evaluation of three-dimensional imaging in laparoscopy. *Gastrointest Endosc* 44:262-267, 1996.

4. Mohr FW, Falk V, Diegeler A, et al: Minimally invasive port-access mitral valve surgery. *J Thorac Cardiovasc Surg* 115:567-576, 1998.
5. Chitwood WR Jr: State of the art review: Videoscopic minimally invasive mitral valve surgery. Trekking to a total endoscopic operation. *Heart Surgery Forum* 1:13-16, 1998.
6. Mack MJ, Acuff TE, Casimir-Ahn H, et al: Video-assisted coronary bypass grafting on the beating heart. *Ann Thorac Surg* 63:S100-S103, 1997.
7. Shennib H, Bastawisy A, McLoughlin J, et al: Robotic computer-assisted telemanipulation enhances coronary artery bypass. *J Thorac Cardiovasc Surg* 117:310-313, 1999.
8. Sackier JM, Wang Y: Robotically assisted laparoscopic surgery. *Surg Endosc* 8:63-66, 1994.
9. Kavoussi LR, Moore RG, Adams JB, et al: Comparison of robotic versus human laparoscopic camera control. *J Urol* 6:2134-2136, 1995.
10. Geis WP, Kim HC, McAfee PC, et al: Synergistic benefits of combined technologies in complex, minimally invasive surgical procedures: Clinical experience and educational processes. *Surg Endosc* 10:1025-1028, 1996.
11. Falk V, Walther T, Autschbach R, et al: Robot-assisted minimally invasive solo mitral valve operation. *J Thorac Cardiovasc Surg* 115:470-471, 1998.
12. Reichenspurner H, Boehm DH, Welz A, et al: 3D-Video– and robot-assisted minimally invasive ASD closure using the port-access techniques. *Heart Surgery Forum* 1:104-106, 1998.
13. Schurr MO, Breitwieser H, Melzer A, et al: Experimental telemanipulation in endoscopic surgery. *Surg Laparosc Endosc* 6:167-175, 1996.
14. Urban V, Wapler M, Neugebauer J, et al: Robot-assisted surgery system with kinesthetic feedback. *Computer Aided Surgery* 3:205-209, 1998.
15. Ducko CT, Stephenson ER Jr, Sankholkar S, et al: Robotically-assisted coronary artery bypass surgery: Moving toward a completely endoscopic procedure. *Heart Surgery Forum* 2:29-37, 1999.
16. Falk V, Gummert J, Walther T, et al: Quality of computer enhanced totally endoscopic coronary bypass graft anastomosis: Comparison to conventional technique. *Eur J Cardiothorac Surg,* in press.
17. Bowersox JC: Telepresence surgery. *Br J Surg* 83:433-434, 1996.
18. Garcia-Ruiz A, Smedira NG, Loop FD, et al: Robotic surgical instruments for dexterity enhancement in thoracoscopic coronary artery bypass graft. *J Laparoendosc Adv Surg Tech* 7:277-283, 1997.
19. Falk V, McLoughlin J, Guthart G, et al: Dexterity enhancement in endoscopic surgery by a computer controlled mechanical wrist. *Minimally Invasive Therapy and Allied Technology,* in press.
20. Green PS, Piantanida TA, Hill JW, et al: Telepresence dexterous procedures in a virtual operating field. *Am Surg* 57:92A, 1992.
21. Bowersox JC, Shah A, Jensen J, et al: Vascular applications of telepresence surgery: Initial feasibility studies in swine. *J Vasc Surg* 23:281-287, 1996.
22. Bowersox JC, Cordts PR, LaPorta AJ: Use of an intuitive telemanipu-

lator system for remote trauma surgery: An experimental study. *J Am Coll Surg* 186:615-621, 1998.

23. Shennib H, Bastawisy A, Mack MJ, et al: Computer-assisted telemanipulation: An enabling technology for endoscopic coronary artery bypass. *Ann Thorac Surg* 66:1060-1063, 1998.

24. Stephenson ER Jr, Sankholkar S, Ducko CT, et al: Robotically assisted microsurgery for endoscopic coronary artery bypass grafting. *Ann Thorac Surg* 66:1064-1067, 1998.

25. Stephenson ER Jr, Sankholkar S, Ducko CT, et al: Successful endoscopic coronary artery bypass grafting: An acute large animal trial. *J Thorac Cardiovasc Surg* 116:1071-1073, 1998.

26. Loulmet D, Carpentier A, d'Attellis N, et al: Endoscopic coronary artery bypass grafting with the aid of robotic assisted instruments. *J Thorac Cardiovas Surg* 118:4-10, 1999.

27. Mohr F: Presented at the 2nd Annual Meeting of the International Society for Minimally Invasive Cardiac Surgery, Paris, May 20-22, 1999.

28. Schüler S: Personal communication.

29. Reichenspurner H, Damiano RJ, Mack M, et al: Experimental and first clinical use of the voice-controlled and computer-assisted surgical system Zeus for endoscopic coronary artery bypass grafting. *J Thorac Cardiovasc Surg* 118:11-16, 1999.

30. Wismer J-M: Vista and robotics: New technologies, new frontiers. *Perfusion* 13:273-277, 1998.

CHAPTER 4

Transplantation for Congenital Heart Disease

Jonah Odim, MD, PhD
Assistant Professor of Surgery, Division of Cardiothoracic Surgery, UCLA School of Medicine, Los Angeles, California

Hillel Laks, MD
Professor and Chief, Division of Cardiothoracic Surgery; Director, Heart and Heart–Lung Transplant Program, UCLA Medical Center, Los Angeles, California

Caron Burch, RN, MSN
Division of Cardiothoracic Surgery, UCLA School of Medicine, Los Angeles, California

Christopher Komanapalli, BS
Medical Student, UCLA School of Medicine, Los Angeles, California

Juan C. Alejos, MD
Assistant Professor of Pediatrics, Division of Pediatric Cardiology, UCLA School of Medicine, Los Angeles, California

T he outcome and acceptance of transplantation for congenital structural anomalies of the heart has lagged considerably behind that for other nonstructural cardiomyopathic etiologies. This marked difference relates to the predilection and concentration of these structural abnormalities in a subpopulation that possesses unique biology notable for a maturing immunologic milieu, hyperplasia and hypertrophy of growth, neuroendocrine and hormonal changes associated with puberty, susceptibility to particular infections, and the potential for long life expectancy. Each of the above phenomena, unique to the pediatric subpopulation, exacts its own price in face of current immunosuppression regimens. Finally, though largely overcome, there were technical challenges related to orthotopic allograft implantation in the face of anomalies of situs, systemic and pulmonary venous connection, great artery morphology, and multiple palliative surgical interventions.

BACKGROUND

Ironically, in 1967, while Barnard[1] was carrying out the seminal human-to-human heart transplantation in Capetown in an adult, Kantrowitz et al,[2] in New York a few days later and with much less fanfare, unsuccessfully implanted the heart from an anencephalic human donor to a 17-day-old infant with Ebstein's anomaly, thereby igniting worldwide a flurry of clinical cardiac transplantation activity. The explosive enthusiasm after the success in South Africa was soon tempered by poor clinical outcomes heralded by primitive immunosuppressive regimens and the ravages of rejection and infection. The early prohibitive morbidity and mortality of orthotopic cardiac transplantation stymied the growth of this therapeutic modality for end-stage heart disease until the decade of the 1980s, with cyclosporine sparking a revival of clinical activity and improved outcomes for heart transplantation.[3,4] Pioneering contributions and perseverance from Lower and Shumway[5] in surgical technique and early transplantation biology, the introduction of a reliable and safe myocardial biopsy technique by Caves et al,[6] and the diagnosis and grading of cardiac rejection by Billingham[7-9] fueled the resurgence of clinical heart transplantation (Tables 1 and 2).

The relative scarcity of infant donor hearts, the immaturity of the neonatal immune system, and the successful results of cardiac

---

TABLE 1.

Stanford Classification for Grading Cardiac Transplant Rejection

Mild rejection	Interstitial and endocardial edema. Few perivascular, pyroninophilic lymphoblasts. Pyroninophilia of endothelial cells.
Moderate rejection	Moderate interstitial infiltrate of pyroninophilic lymphoblasts. Early focal myocyte damage.
Severe rejection	Interstitial infiltrate of neutrophils and lymphoblasts, hemorrhage, myocyte and vascular necrosis.

(Courtesy of Billingham ME: Some recent advances in cardiac pathology. *Hum Pathol* 10:367-386, 1979.)

TABLE 2.
The International Grading System for Cardiac Transplant Rejection

Grade 0	No rejection
Grade 1	A = focal (perivascular or interstitial) infiltrate without necrosis
	B = diffuse but sparse infiltrate without necrosis
Grade 2	One focus only with aggressive infiltration and/or focal myocyte damage
Grade 3	A = multifocal aggressives infiltrates and/or myocyte damage
	B = diffuse inflammatory process with necrosis
Grade 4	Diffuse aggressive polymorphous ± infiltrate, ± edema, ± hemorrhage, ± vasculitis, with necrosis

(Courtesy of Billingham ME, Cary NRB, Hammond ME, et al: A working formulation for the standardization of nomenclature in the diagnosis of heart and lung rejection: Heart rejection study group. *J Heart Transplant* 9:587-593, 1990.)

transplantation in newborn animal models led to the xenotransplantation experiment and the baboon to human transplant in a neonate with hypoplastic left heart syndrome by Bailey et al[10] in Loma Linda in 1985. After a maelstrom of debate in public and medical forums over medico-ethical concerns, Bailey and his group[11-14] pioneered cardiac allotransplantation in the neonatal population—in particular—as primary therapy for hypoplastic left heart syndrome instead of the staged surgical reconstructive procedures advocated by Norwood and his associates. The latter part of the decade of the 1980s witnessed an escalation in the number of pediatric heart transplantation centers and the number of pediatric heart transplants performed worldwide.

Since 1982, based on reports from the registry of the International Society of Heart and Lung Transplantation, there have been more than 3857 heart transplants in the pediatric population, representing 9% to 10% of all heart transplants worldwide.[15,16] The annual volume (about 375) of pediatric heart transplants has remained stable for the last 5 years; however, the downward trend in the number of centers reporting data underlies the forces of regionalization that are concentrating this expertise at fewer centers.[16]

This chapter will review the current approach to heart transplantation in children with congenital heart disease. Patients with either severe congenital cardiac abnormalities or cardiomyopathy secondary to residual or recurrent sequelae from reparative or palliative procedures for structural abnormalities constitute an important growing proportion of the pediatric population that may benefit from organ replacement.

RECIPIENT ISSUES
INDICATIONS FOR CARDIAC TRANSPLANTATION

The major indication for heart transplantation in the infant group (<1 year) remains congenital heart disease in three fourths of cases (Table 3). Allograft replacement for cardiomyopathy plays a minor role in the first year of life. By contrast, for recipients between 1 and 10 years of age (transition age group), the initial increase in congenital heart disease as an indication for transplantation has tapered and plateaued at under 40%, with cardiomyopathy accounting for slightly more than 50% of cases. Retransplantations account for 4% of transplantations in the transition age group. The indication for transplantation in the adolescent group (11-17 years) mirrors that for the adult population, as cardiomyopathy was the indication in 65% of cases and congenital heart disease was the indication in 25% of cases.[16]

TABLE 3.
Indications for Transplantation in Congenital Heart Disease

HLHS
Aortic stenosis with LV endocardial fibroelastosis
Unbalanced AV canal with LV hypoplasia
HLHS equivalent
    TA, D-TGA, RV and aortic hypoplasia
    Single ventricle with aortic hypoplasia
    L-TGA with single ventricle and heart block
Cardiac tumors (rhabdomyomas, fibromas)
Dilated cardiomyopathy
Restrictive cardiomyopathy
Ischemic cardiomyopathy (anomalous origin of the left coronary
  artery)
Intractable arrhythmias
Failed reconstructive and palliative operations with acquired
  myopathy (Mustard, Senning)

Abbreviations: HLHS, Hypoplastic left heart syndrome; LV, left ventricle; RV, right ventricle; AV, atrioventricular; TA, tricuspid atresia; D-TGA, dextro-transposition of the great arteries; L-TGA, levo-transposition of the great arteries.

TABLE 4.
Critical Hemodynamic Data

$$PVRI\ (units/m^2) = \frac{PAP\ (mm\ Hg) - PACWP\ (mm\ Hg)}{CI\ (L/min/m^2)}$$

$$TPG\ (mm\ Hg) = PAP\ (mm\ Hg) - PACWP\ (mm\ Hg)$$

Abbreviations: PVRI, Pulmonary vascular resistance index; *PAP,* mean pulmonary artery pressure; *PACWP,* mean pulmonary artery capillary wedge pressure; *CI,* cardiac index; *TPG,* transpulmonary gradient.

In the UCLA pediatric transplantation experience (117 transplants in 105 patients), an equal number of patients have undergone allograft replacement for dilated cardiomyopathy and congenital heart disease (44% and 42%, respectively). Additional indications in our experience have included arrhythmias, anthracycline toxicity, muscular dystrophy, and restrictive cardiomyopathy. Retransplantation for graft failure represents 8.3% of our 117 transplant cases.

CONTRAINDICATIONS FOR CARDIAC TRANSPLANTATION
Contraindications to pediatric cardiac transplantation due largely to the potential for graft right ventricular failure include an irreversible pulmonary vascular resistance index greater than 6 that is not lowered by inotropy, vasodilatation, and afterload reduction with milrinone, nitroglycerin, prostaglandins, oxygen, dobutamine, or inhaled nitric oxide. Similarly, a persistently elevated transpulmonary gradient of more than 15 mm Hg makes orthotopic heart transplantation prohibitive (Table 4). The most important risk factor for death shortly after heart transplantation is high pulmonary vascular resistance unresponsive to vasodilator therapy. Additional potential contraindications are similar to those for adult cardiac transplantation (Table 5).

PRETRANSPLANT MANAGEMENT
The unique biology of infants with congenital heart disease and major structural abnormalities requires medical strategies that differ from those used for most adult cardiac transplant patients and patients with severe cardiomyopathy. Systemic and coronary perfusion is ductus dependent in many potential recipients of a cardiac allograft. Because the pulmonary and systemic vascular beds are in parallel, not in series, optimal organ perfusion is dependent

TABLE 5.

Contraindications to Transplantation for Congenital
Heart Disease

Irreversible PVRI > 6 units/m^2
Irreversible TPG > 15 mm Hg
Active infection and sepsis
Severe metabolic disease
Severe hepatic dysfunction
Active malignancy (except primary brain tumor)
Multiple congenital anomalies
Advanced multiple organ failure
Socioeconomic factors (noncompliance)

Abbreviations: PVRI, Pulmonary vascular resistance index; *TPG,*
transpulmonary gradient.

on the delicate balance between pulmonary and systemic circulation. Patients with single-ventricle pathophysiology, in whom
maintenance of an unrestrictive atrial septal defect and controlled
patency of the ductus arteriosus are paramount, account for a significant majority of the preoperative mortality of infants on the
pediatric transplant rolls. This mortality may reach as high as 25%
in some settings.

These infants may require mechanical ventilation to regulate
partial pressure of oxygen (Pao$_2$) and carbon dioxide (Paco$_2$)
(hence pulmonary vascular resistance); prostaglandins to maintain
patency of the ductus arteriosus; and sodium bicarbonate and
inotropic drugs for resuscitation en route to a pulmonary-to-sys-
temic blood flow ratio of 1 or less. The degree of restriction at the
foramen ovale will promote increased pulmonary vascular resistance—potentially beneficial in the setting of compromised systemic perfusion. On the other hand, blade or balloon septostomy
is undertaken in the setting of pulmonary venous congestion. In
some instances, children may require an early palliative bridge to
transplantation; for example, a stage one Norwood procedure for
hypoplastic left heart syndrome, or pulmonary artery banding for
univentricular physiology and too much pulmonary blood flow. In
dire straits, with profound pump failure and inadequate oxygen
delivery despite medical and pharmacologic therapy, venoarterial
bypass (extracorporeal membrane oxygenation [ECMO]) and ventricular assist devices can mechanically bridge patients to successful transplantation.[17,18] Diastolic counterpulsation with an

intra-aortic balloon pump plays no clinical role in neonates and infants with end-stage heart failure because of size considerations.

DONOR ISSUES

The success of a pediatric cardiac transplantation program demands careful scrutiny and selection of potential cadaver donors. The growing divergence in donor supply relative to burgeoning recipient demand requires a screening process tailored to specific recipient needs. This flexible clinical approach spurs efficient use of donor organs with minimal wastage of a scare commodity and widens the potential therapeutic benefit.

There are three phases of donor selection.[19] The primary screening is performed by the OPO (organ procurement organization). Pertinent demographic information about the potential donor includes age, height, weight, gender, ABO blood group, mechanism of death, hospital course, and routine laboratory and serologic data. After verification of brain death and informed consent, potential recipients are identified through an extensive computerized database maintained by the United Network Of Organ Sharing (UNOS).

The secondary screening involves notifying the recipient hospital team (the transplant coordinator, cardiac surgeon, and/or cardiologist) that scrutinizes the potential donor, examining past medical history, clinical and hemodynamic status, serology, complete blood cell counts, Gram stains and cultures, arterial blood gas analysis, chest roentgenograms (obtaining specific measurements in the event of important donor-recipient size mismatch), electrocardiograms, echocardiograms (resting or under dobutamine stress), and cineangiograms. This team identifies potential contraindications (absolute and relative) to transplantation and coordinates the clinical management of the donor. Assessment of any adverse issues is always considered in relation to the clinical needs of the potential recipients. A team may be dispatched to the donor hospital to complete this formal evaluation and stabilize a complicated patient.[19]

The final phase or definitive screening occurs at the time of harvest. On arrival at the donor hospital, the cardiothoracic surgeon examines the patient and reviews the medical records, chest roentgenograms (exchanging dimensions from the x-ray with the recipient surgeon), electrocardiograms, echocardiograms, and cineangiograms. Once in the operating room, the surgeon inspects the heart directly looking for signs of myocardial contusion, infarction, and ventricular dysfunction. The great arteries are palpated for thrills and signs of valvular dysfunction or intracardiac shunts.

The coronary arteries are palpated for plaques and gross calcifications—potential harbingers of underlying atherosclerotic occlusive disease. A mini-catherization can be obtained by direct measurement of cardiac chamber, aortic, and main pulmonary artery pressures. If necessary, oximetry can be performed to evaluate intracardiac shunts. The recipient hospital is notified of the findings in the field, and procurement can proceed if indicated. This is usually a multiorgan harvest with several surgical teams from different hospitals. The cardiothoracic surgeon coordinates the operative management of the patient and the sequence of organ retrieval.[19]

The upper cold ischemia limit of the heart has historically been set at 4 to 6 hours. Current organ preservation techniques have extended heart preservation from 6 to 8 hours. The upper limit is particularly true to infant donor procurement and preservation. This biological constraint has limited the geographic area from which donor hearts can be harvested for specific transplant centers and any potential benefit that may accrue from prospective cross-matching potential donor hearts for transplantation. The successful preservation of other solid organs for up to 2 days by flushing the organs with the University of Wisconsin (UW) solution and storage at hypothermia (0°C to 5°C) has led to the substitution of UW solution for the Stanford solution in our heart transplantation program.[19,20] Cellular impermeable agents (eg, lactobionic acid, raffinose, and hydroxyethyl starch) prevent cell swelling during cold ischemic storage. The addition of glutathione and adenosine may promote organ recovery by combating the reperfusion injury caused by free radicals, and stimulating high-energy phosphate replenishment. Donor cardiectomy is performed after diastolic arrest and flush cooling of the empty heart with cold UW solution and topical saline slush. In the case of transplantation for complex congenital heart disease with structural anomalies, it is paramount to bring extensive donor tissue including the aortic arch vessels and descending aorta, the branch pulmonary arteries, the superior caval vein in continuity with the innominate vein, and the pericardium. Our current protocol requires infusion of UW solution (10-12 mL/kg) at a mean aortic root pressure of 40 to 50 mm Hg for 4 to 6 minutes for infant donors, and 60 to 70 mm Hg over a similar time course for large adolescent and adult donors. The excised allograft is rinsed in cold UW solution to remove blood and submerged in cold UW solution before placement in sterile bowel bags for transportation in a chest of ice. At the recipient hospital, orthotopic transplantation is performed using a bicaval technique in situs solitus recipient hearts with concordant connections and cardiomyopathy. If the caval veins are particularly small or there is important caval size mismatch and other major structural abnormalities, the traditional atrial cuff anastomotic technique may be used with continuous topical endocardial cold plasmalyte solution infusion. All allografts are reperfused with leukocyte-depleted aspartate-glutamate–enriched warm blood cardioplegia for 4 minutes, followed by 4 minutes of leukocyte-depleted warm blood before releasing the aortic cross-clamp. Our experience with the use of UW solution and leukocyte-depleted reperfusion has reduced the incidence of allograft failure associated with long donor ischemia times (>5 hours).

SIZE MISMATCH

Earlier guidelines established that heart transplantation is safely performed when donor-recipient size mismatch is greater than 0.8 in the setting of normal recipient pulmonary vascular resistance and transpulmonary gradient. A donor is considered marginal if mismatch is less than 0.7 or if body surface area of donor and recipient differ by more than 30%. Before accepting an undersized donor heart, other variables in both donor and recipient should be considered, such as duration of donor ischemic time, lean body mass, recipient's pulmonary artery pressures, donor heart hypertrophy, and gender mismatch, particularly when considering implanting an undersized female heart into a male recipient. The goal is to match the donor myocardial mass to the circulatory demands of the recipient. In this context, an estimation of lean body mass is more relevant than absolute weight, particularly in obesity. Most patients with end-stage heart failure have cardiomegaly and can accept a larger donor heart. This is particularly true for neonatal and infant recipients for whom size-matched donor organs are more difficult to come by. A greater discrepancy in size match (donor-to-recipient ratios of 3:1 to 5:1) is generally tolerated, sometimes requiring removal of recipient costal cartilages to enlarge the mediastinal domain for an oversized allograft. Undersizing should be avoided whenever possible, particularly in patients with elevated pulmonary vascular resistance and reoperative sternotomy (higher likelihood for blood transfusion), because there is insufficient time for myocardial remodeling and acclimation, and the incidence of postoperative acute right-sided heart failure is high. In the pediatric age range where potential for discrepant size mismatch between donor and recipient exists, additional evaluation includes donor-to-recipient ratios of dimensions from the chest roentgenogram; namely, the distances of aortic knob to apex, right lung apex to diaphragm, and the largest transverse diameter of the myocardial mass are helpful.

OPERATIVE TECHNIQUES FOR MAJOR CARDIAC STRUCTURAL MALFORMATIONS

Donor organ procurement is guided by the specific anatomical requirements for the recipient. In the case of cardiomyopathy with normal situs and atrioventricular and ventricular-arterial concordance, the technique of harvest mimics that for the typical adult recipient. Patients with congenital heart disease heralded by structural abnormalities require extra and judicious donor graft procurement to permit bicaval or atrial orthotopic implantation.[21-26] In circumstances where biological tissue is lacking, we have successfully used synthetic conduits to permit unencumbered orthotopic transplantation. Four distinct anatomical issues require the attention of both donor and recipient surgeon; namely, abnormalities of situs, main and branch pulmonary artery, ascending aorta and arch, and systemic and pulmonary venous connection. Certain instances may call for procuring donor superior vena cava in continuity with the innominate bridging vein, ascending aorta, arch, and descending aorta, and donor pericardium along with the cardiac organ to enable engrafting and unobstructed systemic and pulmonary venous pathways. Creative planning and surgical execution allow successful orthotopic transplantation of virtually all complex congenital structural abnormalities of the heart. In addition, we have successfully used donor allografts with congenital malformations—atrial septal defects and repaired total anomalous pulmonary venous return—in pediatric recipients.

There is some experience with heterotopic cardiac transplantation in children at high risk for standard orthotopic transplantation, specifically, those with elevated pulmonary vascular resistance. Fourteen children with cardiomyopathy between the ages of 15 months and 16 years have undergone a piggyback transplantation with the donor allograft in a heterotopic position biologically assisting the recipient left heart.[27] In this series, Radley-Smith et al report an early hospital mortality of 14% with the 12 survivors at a mean follow-up period of 46 months (range, 4-87 months) receiving cyclosporine and azathioprine immunosuppression. The survivors have normal exercise tolerance, and a year after transplantation the pulmonary vascular resistance has decreased to the normal range. Actuarial survival is 70.5% at 3 and 5 years.[27]

Although left ventricular assist devices are used successfully to bridge failing hearts in adults and large children to transplantation, long-term mechanical cardiac devices for smaller infants (body surface area < 1.5 m^2) are not yet available.

POSTOPERATIVE MANAGEMENT

The denervated pediatric allograft requires the maintenance of chronotropic support with drugs or atrial pacing. In addition, because the major cause of primary graft failure relates to right ventricular failure secondary to increased pulmonary vascular resistance, vigilance in prevention with judicious transfusion of homologous blood products and volume, and aggressive afterload reduction with agents including milrinone, prostaglandin E$_1$, nitrates, prostacyclin, and inhaled nitric oxide may prevent this potentially irreversible state. Occasionally, mechanical afterload reduction of the pulmonary circulation may be necessary using a right ventricular assist device or ECMO. For children in whom synthetic grafts or conduits were used to complete orthotopic transplantation, anticoagulation with warfarin for a year is the practice at UCLA.

IMMUNOSUPPRESSION

The immunosuppression regimen consists of triple-drug therapy with cyclosporine A, azathioprine, and corticosteroids in many centers.[20,28-30] For the first 6 postoperative months, the therapeutic range of blood cyclosporine A levels is 250 to 300 ng/mL. This target level is reduced to 100 to 200 ng/mL thereafter.

More recently, tacrolimus (FK 506) has been used instead of cyclosporine A in some pediatric patients. We have witnessed improved outcomes in high-risk recipients, in particular, children with congenital heart disease. Our criteria for the use of tacrolimus immunotherapy include the presence of congenital heart defects, failure to respond to cyclosporine A, and a history of blood transfusion. Cytolytic therapy with monoclonal or polyclonal antibody preparations is usually reserved for recurrent or refractory rejection; however, some centers use rabbit antithymocyte globulin or T cell–specific murine antibody OKT3 for initial induction therapy or in patients with important perioperative renal dysfunction. The Pediatric Heart Transplant Study Group has studied the controversial issue of safety and efficacy of induction immunotherapy with antithymocyte preparations.[31] The outcomes of two groups who received either OKT3 (n = 101) or rabbit polyclonal antithymocyte sera (n = 105) and 255 recipients who did not receive antithymocyte antibodies demonstrated an important reduction in late deaths in recipients younger than 6 months, while not being associated with higher rates of infectious or malignant complications at a follow-up period of 36 months.[31] In their multi-institutional study, polyclonal antithymocyte sera was superior to monoclonal OKT3 with respect to graft and patient survival. The multi-institutional nature of the study, center variation, and clinical decision-making are obvious limitations to this study.

Corticosteroids may result in long-term morbidity in children after heart transplantation. These complications include obesity, hypertension, hyperlipidemia, osteoporosis, cataracts, peptic ulcer disease, and growth retardation. Thus, every attempt is made to wean corticosteroids after the initial 6 months posttransplantation. In many instances these patients will remain immunologically stable on double-drug therapy.[20]

Mycophenolate mofetil inhibits the *de novo* pathway for purine biosynthesis and decreases rejection in animal and human models of allotransplantation. We have substituted this drug for azathioprine in a few of our pediatric cardiac transplant patients with favorable results. The effects of the drug enhance those of cyclosporine because of action later in the lymphocyte activation pathway. Mycophenolate appears effective in refractory biopsy-proven rejection of cardiac allografts under triple-drug immunosuppression. A report from Toronto regarding the use of mycophenolate mofetil in 21 pediatric heart transplant recipients confirms the effectiveness of this modality in rejection treatment and primary rejection prophylaxis, with tolerable side effects, allowing children to wean off steroids.[32]

Hypercholesterolemia is common after cardiac transplantation and is associated with the development of transplant coronary artery disease, which limits long-term patient and graft survival.[33] The lowering of serum cholesterol levels is associated with the regression of atherosclerotic disease in patients with coronary atherosclerosis who are not transplant candidates. Pravastatin, a hydrophilic hepatic hydroxymethylglutaryl coenzyme A reductase inhibitor, dramatically reduces serum cholesterol levels in patients after heart transplantation. In an open-labeled randomized trial of 97 heart transplant patients, besides an important and significant reduction in serum cholesterol levels, the pravastatin-treated group also had less frequent cardiac rejection accompanied by hemodynamic compromise, better survival, and a lower incidence of transplant coronary artery disease.[33] The mechanism of this effect is via reduction in natural killer cell cytotoxicity and enhanced immunosuppression. These findings in our adult cardiac transplantation experience have led us to administer oral pravastatin to our pediatric transplant recipients.

Monitoring for rejection requires clinical, echocardiographic, and endomyocardial biopsy assessment in the child. Endomyocardial biopsy provides the definitive diagnosis. Clinical, electrocardiographic, and echocardiographic methods, although noninvasive, lack sensitivity and specificity for the diagnosis of rejection. Clinical assessment includes the evaluation of temperature, blood pressure, heart rate and rhythm, and changes in the child's well-being and appetite. R-wave summation electrocardiography may heighten suspicion for acute rejection. Increases in left ventricular dimensions (including left ventricular end-diastolic dimension, left ventricular posterior wall thickness) and a decrease in left ventricular shortening fraction may portend a lymphocytic infiltrative process and accompanying edema consistent with rejection. Other signs of potential rejection include a new pericardial effusion and new-onset mitral regurgitation. Endomyocardial biopsy provides material for assessment of acute and humoral/vascular rejection and remains the "gold standard" for the diagnosis of acute rejection after cardiac transplantation (Tables 1 and 2). There is a paucity of data supporting guidelines for the use of routine surveillance biopsies in pediatric cardiac transplant recipients.[34,35] A recent study from Minnesota, and supported by the practice at other centers, demonstrates that episodes of acute rejection are relatively uncommon while patients are receiving triple-drug immunosuppression. Surveillance endomyocardial biopsies in the first 6 months postoperatively may show unsuspected rejection; however, routine surveillance biopsies more than 6 months after cardiac transplantation are unlikely to show rejection in the absence of signs, symptoms, and other test results.[35]

REJECTION

The majority of acute cellular rejection episodes occur within the first 6 months after transplantation, with clustering in the initial 3 months. Pulse administration of high-dose intravenous steroids (methylprednisolone) is used as initial treatment for a diagnosed episode of acute rejection. Rejection accompanied by hemodynamic compromise may require additional aggressive therapy with cytolytic therapy or methotrexate. Steroid-resistant cardiac rejection is treated with tacrolimus or mycophenolate mofetil, or photopheresis in the older patient. A diagnosis of humoral rejection requires prevention of B-cell production of antibody with cyclophosphamide, plasmapheresis, and intravenous heparin.[20]

RESULTS

Children are subject to the same postoperative complications that occur in adults undergoing heart transplantation. However, in recipients with unique structural abnormalities requiring complex reconstructive techniques at the time of allograft implantation, occasional obstruction of systemic and pulmonary venous pathways, branch pulmonary arteries, and aortic arch can occur. The tracheobronchial tree is also subject to compression.

Transplantation of a large donor heart into a relatively small recipient may cause systemic hypertension in the neonate or infant in the immediate postoperative period. This can result in mental status changes and cerebrovascular accidents, including coma and seizures, thus mandating aggressive control of blood pressure with β-blockers and vasodilators and the avoidance of alkalosis in patients with important size mismatch.

Growth retardation is observed in pediatric recipients of heart allografts. Risk factor analysis for inappropriate growth after heart transplantation in 44 pediatric heart transplant survivors showed growth rates for height are reduced more than growth rates for weight. Transplantation at older age, and severe (grade > 3) or frequent episodes of rejection requiring high-dose steroid pulses are significant risk factors for decreased growth.[36]

The Pediatric Heart Transplant Study Group has recently attempted to estimate the time-related cause-specific mortality after pediatric heart transplantation from a multi-institutional group of 680 pediatric heart transplants. In their analysis, rejection and infection remain the most likely causes of death during the first 5 years after pediatric cardiac transplantation, with the exception of recipients with the diagnosis of hypoplastic left heart syndrome in whom early graft failure was the culprit. Thus, strategies to prevent early graft failure in this subpopulation would impact favorably on long-term survival. For the rest of pediatric recipients of cardiac allografts, strategies to improve rejection monitoring, prevent rejection, and improve current immunosuppression may reduce late mortality and morbidity from rejection and infection.

At our institution, pediatric heart transplantation has become standard therapy for terminal heart failure, assuming a suitable donor allograft is available. Since 1984, 105 children aged 15 days to 18 years (mean, 9.3 years) underwent 117 orthotopic heart transplantations. There were 11 (9.4%) retransplantations. Indications for transplantation were dilated cardiomyopathy (44.4%), congenital heart disease (41.0%), graft failure (6.8%), and other (6.9%). Immunosuppression consisted of cyclosporine A or tacrolimus-based triple-drug therapy (with azathioprine and prednisone). Univariate analysis identified mean donor-to-recipient weight ratio, mean follow-up time, UNOS status 1, perioperative ECMO, donor sex, and donor race as significant ($P < .05$) between patients that were alive versus dead or with graft loss. Multivariate Cox analysis demonstrated that donor-to-recipient weight ratio, the presence of a mechanical assist device, donor ischemic time, cardiopulmonary bypass time, recipient cross-clamp time, and perioperative ECMO were independent predictors for risk of death or graft failure. Number of rejection episodes ranged from 0 to 7. One-month, 6-month, 1-year, and 5-year patient survival after transplantation was 90%, 81%, 80%, and 56.8%, respectively, with a mean follow-up of 33.5 months (range, 1 day to 164 months). Among the primary transplantation group of 105 patients, early death occurred in 12 patients (11.4%), and late death occurred in 18 of the 93 remaining transplant recipients (19.4%). Of the 11 retransplantation recipients, early death occurred in 1 patient (9.1%), and late death occurred in 2 of the remaining 10 patients (20%).

Elective cardiac retransplantation can be performed with acceptable morbidity and mortality. Between 1985 and 1998, 18 of 332 children (primary transplantation) have undergone cardiac retransplantation at Loma Linda at a median age of 7.1 years (range, 52 days to 18.8 years).[37] Indications for retransplantation were allograft vasculopathy (13 patients), primary graft failure (4), and acute rejection (1). Median interval to retransplantation was 5.8 years (range, 10 days to 9.4 years), with an operative mortality of 16.7%. There was 1 late death from severe rejection. Actuarial survival for the retransplantation group was 77.8% ± 9.8% compared with 71.3% ± 2.6% for the primary transplantation group (P = NS). The rejection rate for the first 6 months after retransplantation was 0.85% compared with 0.79% for the primary grafting.[37]

SUMMARY

Refinements in surgical technique, donor and recipient myocardial preservation, and immunosuppression have brought pediatric heart transplantation for end-stage heart failure (whatever the cause) from the heyday of clinical experimentation to the realm of a viable therapeutic. Heart transplantation in this subpopulation yields excellent early and midterm survival. Acute rejection remains an important cause of morbidity and mortality after heart transplantation in children. Future improvement in quality of life for these patients calls for newer immunosuppressive strategies to reduce acute rejection episodes and ultimately improve long-term graft survival.

REFERENCES

1. Barnard CN: A human cardiac transplant: An interim report of a successful operation performed at Groote Schuur Hospital, Capetown. *S Afr Med J* 41:1271-1274, 1967.
2. Kantrowitz A, Haller JD, Joos H, et al: Transplantation of the heart in an infant and an adult. *Am J Cardiol* 22:782-790, 1968.
3. Borel JF: Immunosuppressive properties of cyclosporine A (CyA). *Transplant Proc* 12:233, 1980.
4. Kahan BD: Cyclosporine. *N Engl J Med* 321:1725-1738, 1989.
5. Lower RR, Shumway NE: Studies on orthotopic homotransplantation of the canine heart. *Surg Forum* 11:18-20, 1960.
6. Caves PK, Stinson EB, Billingham ME, et al: Percutaneous transvenous intravenous endomyocardial biopsy in human heart recipients. *Ann Thorac Surg* 16:325-336, 1973.
7. Billingham ME: Some recent advances in cardiac pathology. *Hum Pathol* 10:367-386, 1979.
8. Billingham ME: Diagnosis of cardiac rejection by endomyocardial biopsy. *J Heart Transplant* 1:25-30, 1982.
9. Billingham ME, Cary NRB, Hammond ME, et al: A working formulation for the standardization of nomenclature in the diagnosis of heart and lung rejection: Heart rejection study group. *J Heart Transplant* 9:587-593, 1990.
10. Bailey LL, Nehlsen-Cannarella SL, Concepcion W, et al: Baboon to human cardiac xenotransplantation in a neonate. *JAMA* 254:3321-3329, 1985.
11. Bailey LL, Concepcion W, Shattuck H, et al: Method of heart transplantation for treatment of hypoplastic left heart syndrome. *J Thorac Cardiovasc Surg* 92:1-5, 1986.
12. Bailey LL, Nehlsen-Cannarella SL, Doroshow RW, et al: Cardiac allotransplantation in newborns as therapy for hypoplastic left heart syndrome. *N Engl J Med* 115:949-951, 1986.
13. Bailey LL, Assaad AN, Trimm F, et al: Orthotopic transplantation during early infancy as therapy for incurable congenital heart disease. *Ann Surg* 208:279-286, 1988.
14. Bailey LL, and the Loma Linda University Pediatric Heart Transplant Group: Bless the babies: One hundred fifteen late survivors of heart transplantation during the first year of life. *J Thorac Cardiovasc Surg* 105:805-815, 1993.
15. Boucek MM, Novick RJ, Bennett LE, et al: The registry of the International Society of Heart and Lung Transplantation: First official pediatric report—1997. *J Heart Lung Transplant* 16:1189-1206, 1997.
16. Boucek MM, Novick RJ, Bennett LE, et al: The registry of the

International Society of Heart and Lung Transplantation: Second official pediatric report—1998. *J Heart Lung Transplant* 17:1141-1160, 1998.

17. Marelli D, Laks H, Amsel B, et al: Temporary mechanical support with the BVS 5000 assist device during treatment of acute myocarditis. *J Card Surg* 12:55-59, 1997.

18. Helman DN, Addonizio LJ, Morales DLS, et al: Implantable left ventricular assist devices can successfully bridge pediatric patients to transplant. *J Heart Lung Transplant* 18:89, 1999.

19. Odim J, Marelli D, Laks H: Cadaver heart donor selection criteria. *American Society of Transplantation: A Primer on Transplantation,* ed 2, in press

20. Kobashigawa JA, Laks H, Marelli D, et al: The University of California at Los Angeles experience in heart transplantation, in Cecka JM, Terasaki PI (eds): *Clinical Transplants 1998.*

21. Chartrand C: Pediatric cardiac transplantation despite atrial and venous return anomalies. *Ann Thorac Surg* 52:716-721, 1991.

22. Doty DB, Renlund DG, Caputo GR, et al: Cardiac transplantation in situs inversus. *J Thorac Cardiovasc Surg* 99:493-499, 1990.

23. Allard M, Assaad A, Bailey LL, et al: Surgical techniques in pediatric heart transplantation. *J Heart Lung Transplant* 10:808-827, 1991.

24. Mayer JE, Perry S, O'Brien P, et al: Orthotopic heart transplantation for complex congenital heart disease. *J Thorac Cardiovasc Surg* 99:484-492, 1990.

25. Vouhe PR, Tamiser D, Le J, et al: Pediatric cardiac transplantation for congenital heart defects: Surgical considerations and results. *Ann Thorac Surg* 56:1239-1247, 1993.

26. Menkis AH, and The Paediatric Heart Transplant Group: Expanding applicability of transplantation after multiple prior palliative procedures. *Ann Thorac Surg* 52:722-726, 1991.

27. Radley-Smith R, Khaghani A, Yacoub M: Medium term results of children with two hearts. *J Heart Lung Transplant* 18:84A, 1999.

28. Fullerton DA, Campbell DN, Jones SD, et al: Heart transplantation in children and young adults: Early and intermediate-term results. *Ann Thorac Surg* 59:804-812, 1995.

29. Pennington DG, Noedel N, McBride LR, et al: Heart transplantation in children: An international survey. *Ann Thorac Surg* 52:710-715, 1995.

30. Mitchell MB, Campbell DN, Clarke DR, et al: Infant heart transplantation: Improved intermediate results. *J Thorac Cardiovasc Surg* 116:242-252, 1998.

31. Boucek RJ, and the Pediatric Heart Transplant Study Group: Induction immunotherapy in pediatric heart transplant recipients: A multicenter study. *J Heart lung Transplant* 18:460-469, 1999.

32. Dipchand AI, Benson L, McCrindle BW, et al: Mycophenolate mofetil in pediatric heart transplant recipients: A single center experience. *J Heart Lung Transplant* 18:83A-84A, 1999.

33. Kobashigawa JA, Katznelson S, Laks H, et al: Effect of pravastatin on outcomes after cardiac transplantation. *N Engl J Med* 333:621-627, 1995.

34. Balzer DT, Moorhead S, Saffitz JE, et al: Utility of surveillance biopsies in infant heart transplant recipients. *J Heart Lung Transplant* 14:1095-1101, 1995.

35. Braunlin EA, Shumway SJ, Bolman RM, et al: Usefulness of surveillance endomyocardial biopsy after pediatric cardiac transplantation. *Clin Transplant* 3:184-189, 1998.

36. Flaspohler T, Bando K, Caldwell R, et al: Risk factor analysis for inappropriate growth after pediatric heart transplantation (htx). *J Heart Lung Transplant* 18:91A, 1999.

37. Dearani JA, Razzouk AJ, Gundry SR, et al: Pediatric cardiac retransplantation: Experience at a single institution. *J Heart Lung Transplant* 18:70A, 1999.

CHAPTER 5

Surgical Risk Assessment

Fred H. Edwards, MD
Professor of Surgery, University of Florida; Chief, Adult Cardiothoracic
Surgery, University of Florida Health Science Center, Jacksonville,
Florida

Frederick L. Grover, MD
Chief, Department of Surgery, University of Colorado Health Sciences
Center, Denver, Colorado

In recent years, operative risk assessment has come to be an integral part of the practice of cardiothoracic surgery. In spite of this, risk assessment still remains one of the most elusive and misunderstood concepts in our specialty. This is largely because of the statistical detail inherent in most risk assessment techniques and because this type of analysis has only recently become widely accepted. In addition, some surgeons are understandably reluctant to make the intellectual commitment to explore a challenging field that seems to have only an obscure influence on their practice. There seems to be the perception that risk assessment is probably useful, but in ways that remain vague to the average surgeon.

This chapter seeks to clear the fog associated with modern surgical risk assessment. The discussion that follows is directed toward those having little background in biostatistics and is specifically designed to emphasize only the most practical aspects of the field.

THE BIG PICTURE

Consider how we go about the business of traditional risk assessment. We are typically presented with a patient having a myriad of risk factors that are likely to have a bearing on surgical outcome. To make an estimate of operative risk we rely on several sources of information, probably beginning with our personal experience with similar patients. This approach is highly subjective and is all the more difficult because we are unlikely to have a substantial experience with patients exactly like the one at hand. If we want more objective information, we may go to the literature to investigate reported series of patients undergoing similar operations. It then becomes necessary to attempt matching the risk factors of our patient with those in the literature. Although it may be possible to find one or even a few matching risk factors, it is distinctly unlikely that we will find an exact match. Furthermore, even if a close match is found, it may be a leap of faith to extrapolate the experience of that reporting institution to our own hospital. So, after all is said and done, we really guess at the predicted risk. This is hopefully an educated guess, but a guess nevertheless.

This method of risk assessment is certainly not without value and has served us well in the past. Today, however, we need not confine our approach to a process that is totally subjective.

Clearly there is a compelling need for an objective, accurate, reproducible and scientifically valid estimate of risk for an individual patient. Statistical *risk models* are designed to perform exactly this task. A detailed explanation of risk models is presented in the next section, but for now it is useful to regard models in a more general context. At this point, we should recognize that models mathematically manipulate all important patient risk factors to generate a predicted operative risk for a given patient. In other words, the model determines the *net impact* of all risk factors for an individual patient. It is important to recognize that the predicted risk calculated by the model will be dependent on the population of patients used to develop the model.

The New York State Cardiac Surgery Reporting System[1] can be used as an example to clarify these points. This database consists of patients undergoing coronary artery bypass grafting (CABG) and contains numerous risk factors as well as the outcome for each registered patient. Models of this population have been developed to predict the probability of operative death after CABG. For a given patient, the unique array of risk factors is entered into the model and the probability of operative mortality is calculated. As an example, let us say that a predicted risk of 8% is calculated. The following statement is then warranted: "Based on the experience of the New York State Cardiac Surgery Reporting System, of every 100 patients presenting with similar risk factors, 8 would be expected to die after CABG."

Risk models, then, provide us with an *objective* estimate of risk for an *individual* patient. This information can be used in at least three ways: patient counseling, medical decision-making, and outcomes assessment. The first two applications exploit the ability of risk models to be applied to an individual patient, whereas the third application focuses on groups of patients.

The process of outcomes assessment requires some elaboration. For purposes of discussion, we will focus on CABG operative mortality as the "outcome." Assessment of operative outcome necessarily implies a comparison of one set of results with another set of results. Thoracic surgeons have long recognized that operative outcomes cannot be scrutinized solely on the basis of raw operative mortality rates. Before comparing the results of one group with another, it is imperative to ensure that patients of equal risk are being compared. Models provide the objective mechanism for this type of *risk-adjusted* comparison.[2] In general, an appropriate risk model is used to calculate the predicted risk for patients in each group (Fig 1; see color plate I). The patient records in each group are then collated in order of predicted risk and divided into several subsets. This *risk stratification* allows subsets of one group to be compared with the corresponding subset of the other group so that a true "apples to apples" comparison can be made (Fig 2; see color plate I). With these matched subsets, one may then statistically compare the *actual mortality* in each group to determine whether a significant difference exists.

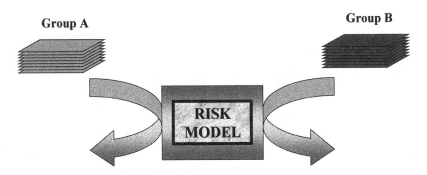

Predicted Risk - Group A		Predicted Risk - Group B	
Patient #287	1%	Patient #459	0.7%
Patient #46	1.5%	Patient #5654	1.1%
Patient #7833	1.6 %	Patient #843	2.6 %

FIGURE 1.
Generation of predicted risk. Data from patient records are entered into the risk model to obtain predicted estimates of operative mortality for each patient. The results are sequentially arranged in order of predicted mortality.

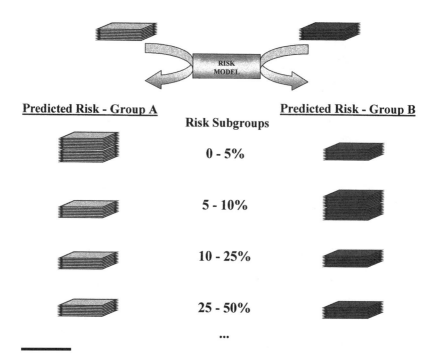

FIGURE 2.

Risk stratification. In each major group, patient records are separated into bins containing patients of approximately equal risk. This allows patients in one group to be directly compared with matched patients of similar risk in the other group.

Interhospital comparisons may be useful, but such analyses do not necessarily allow a comparison with a recognized standard of care. On the other hand, if the population used to derive the risk model is based on an accepted *standard*, then the model becomes a true benchmark. With a model of this kind, it becomes unnecessary to compare results with those of other institutions because the model predicts outcome based on an accepted standard of care. A given institution can conduct an assessment of operative results simply by using the model to stratify a selected group of patients according to predicted risk. The entire group of patients can then be divided into meaningful risk subsets, and the predicted mortality of each subset can be statistically compared with the actual mortality of that subset. The Society of Thoracic Surgeons National Cardiac Surgery Database, commonly called the *STS Database,* uses risk models of this type based on a national experience in cardiac surgery.[3-5]

ANATOMY OF A RISK MODEL

Typically there are three parts to a risk model: the risk factors, the statistical algorithm, and the predicted outcome (Fig 3; see color plate II). For our purposes, we will focus on models used to predict operative outcome associated with cardiac surgery.

OUTCOME

There are numerous outcomes that can be selected, but here we will focus exclusively on operative mortality because that is by far the most common in cardiac surgery models. However, one need not be limited to predicting operative mortality. In fact, there is considerable enthusiasm for developing models that will predict various types of postoperative morbidity, patient length of stay, and hospital cost.[6]

Cardiac surgery risk models are not designed to predict whether a patient will survive or die after surgery. Instead, the *probability* of operative mortality is calculated. This predicted outcome is based on a statistical relationship between patient risk factors and the observed mortality in the population at hand. The predicted mortality reflects the probability of postoperative death for patients having similar comorbidity *based on the experience of the population used to develop the model.*

RISK FACTORS

The risk factors are those preoperative patient characteristics that are thought to influence operative mortality. These factors are necessarily restricted to preoperative findings and should not include intraoperative or postoperative parameters. In most applications, an initial pool of risk factors is subjected to a univariate analysis to determine whether a given parameter is associated with the outcome. Those factors found to be statistically linked with outcome

Risk Factors

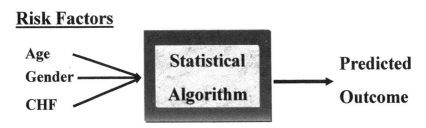

FIGURE 3.
Risk model schematic. *Abbreviation: CHF,* Congestive heart failure.

are then examined by multivariate analysis to determine those factors that are independently associated with operative mortality. Arbitrary constraints are selected to allow for possible entry and eventual retention of risk factors into the model. This selection of constraints is at the discretion of the development team and ideally is strongly influenced by clinical considerations. In models developed by the STS Database team, for example, liberal entry and retention criteria have been used so that a relatively large number of risk factors will be incorporated into the models.

STATISTICAL ALGORITHM

This represents the "brains" of the model and can take several forms. In the final analysis, these algorithms are simply equations which, like all equations, are made up of constants and variables. The constants are derived from the population used to develop the model, whereas the variables represent specific risk factors for the individual patient being evaluated. There are several types of risk equations used in this context.

1. Logistic regression. The most common approach is based on *logistic regression* techniques. Logistic models have gained widespread acceptance, and the methods used to develop them have become fairly standardized.[4,5] In general, the accuracy and reliability of these models have been good. Most commercial statistics software packages contain programs specifically devoted to logistic regression analysis. However, there is some variability in the construction of these models, and different investigators may well produce different models for the same patient population. Usually these differences have only minimal clinical significance, so this is regarded as a relatively minor consideration. A more significant disadvantage is that logistic models must have complete information on all risk factors before outcome calculations can be carried out.

2. Theorem of Bayes. Models based on *Bayesian theory* have also been used with good success in this context.[3] Bayesian models have not gained the popularity of logistic regression models, but they offer some distinct advantages. The development of Bayesian models is more intuitive and straightforward as compared with that of logistic models. Variability is not an issue because each patient population is associated with a unique Bayesian risk equation, whereas several different logistic models may be developed to represent that same population. The selection of risk factors, which is often laborious with logistic models, is easy with Bayesian approaches. Probably the most

significant advantage is that Bayesian models seem to be more forgiving of incomplete data and can produce very acceptable results even when several risk factors are not specified. Unfortunately, few commercial statistics software packages contain programs specifically devoted to the development of Bayesian models.

3. Additive approach. Several *additive methods* have become popular in recent years.[7] Very reasonable accuracy has been obtained for the limited populations in which these models have been applied. These predictive tools are derived from standard statistical methods and are then simplified so that each risk factor is assigned a number representing its relative impact on operative mortality. The predicted mortality for a given patient is then estimated by the sum of the numbers corresponding to the selected risk factors. These additive models offer the advantage of simplicity and the ability to estimate operative mortality without reliance on computer support. Accurate models of this sort can have a real application at the bedside, but when comparing a large population with an accepted benchmark, computer support will almost invariably be necessary.

4. Neural networks. *Neural network* approaches offer some theoretical advantages.[8] These models are based on iterative feedback-and-correction schemes that seem appropriate for the task at hand. In general, as more and more patient characteristics are entered into the model, the neural network progressively "learns" the associations between preoperative patient parameters and postoperative outcome. At this point, there have been very few studies of CABG populations, so it is impossible to assess the reliability of neural models in this area. This process of model development requires extraordinary computer support and special expertise in a particularly complex field of statistical theory. Neural networks may eventually find some role in surgical outcomes assessment, but at present these models are restricted to groups having a special interest and expertise in this field.

The advantages and disadvantages of each algorithm allow one to logically select the most appropriate technique (Table 1). Surprisingly, there appears to be little difference in the accuracy of these models.[9,10] Certainly this observation is debatable, but it does appear that there are no major differences in performance when the models are rigorously derived and are used to predict operative mortality after coronary bypass surgery.

TABLE 1.
Comparative Model Characteristics

	Performance	Ease of Development	Ease of Risk Factor Analysis	Variability	Handling of Incomplete Data	Acceptance
Logistic	++++	++	++	++	+	++++
Bayesian	++++	+++	++++	++++	++++	++
Additive	+++	+++	+++	++	++	+++
Neural network	Unknown	+	++++	+	++++	+

Abbreviations: ++++, excellent; +++, good; ++, acceptable; +, marginal.

EVALUATION OF A MODEL
RISK FACTOR ANALYSIS

A model determines the net impact of all risk factors, but it is often instructive to focus on the significance of individual risk factors. Fortunately, the process of model development lends itself to this type of analysis. In the course of developing any model, patient risk factors are statistically scrutinized for inclusion or exclusion, depending on the influence exerted on outcome.

Logistic regression models typically rely on both univariate and multivariate techniques to determine the statistical importance of each risk factor. The univariate analysis is straightforward and simply determines whether there is a statistically significant difference between the operative mortality of a group of patients with the risk factor as compared with a group without that factor. Often a chi-square analysis is used to make this determination, but other options may be called into play depending on the circumstances. The difference in mortality is mathematically associated with a *P* value, which gives the probability that the difference is caused by chance alone. In most surgical series, a *P* value of less than .05 is considered "significant," indicating that there is a real difference in the groups being compared. As an example, a recent study based on the STS Database experience found that diabetic patients had a CABG operative mortality of 4.1%, whereas those without diabetes had a mortality of 3.0%. The chi-square analysis of these groups yielded a *P* value of less than .005 ($P < .005$), indicating that the observed difference in mortality was almost certainly real and not caused by chance. For that patient population, one concludes that diabetes is a statistically significant risk factor for operative death after CABG.

The univariate analysis allows one to determine whether a certain risk factor is significant, but it provides no information as to how significant it may be. To investigate this, it is useful to associate each risk factor with an *odds ratio*. The odds ratio provides clinically useful information that can be used to better understand the degree to which a risk factor influences prognosis. The odds ratio refers to the odds that a patient with the given risk factor will die after CABG divided by the odds that a patient without the risk factor will die, all other factors being equal. For example, in the 1995 CABG patients registered in the STS Database, the odds ratio associated with preoperative renal failure was 2.0, indicating that patients with renal failure were twice as likely to die after CABG as compared with patients having identical risk except for the absence of renal failure.

Bayesian studies are based on *conditional probabilities*, which also provide useful information about specific risk factors. In general terms, the conditional probability refers to the frequency of an observation given that a certain outcome has occurred. When used in the present context, the conditional probability is the frequency of a risk factor for patients in each outcome group (survival or death). Bayesian models are dependent on a matrix of conditional probabilities that are determined by answering questions of this type: "Of those surviving patients, what fraction had this risk factor?" "Of those that died, what fraction had this risk factor?" This series of questions is answered for each of the selected risk factors to generate a conditional probability matrix, which is then used to represent the constants in the Bayesian equation. Examination of a conditional probability matrix, then, provides valuable information about the relative importance of each risk factor and its association with outcome.[11]

VALIDATION
Validation is the process of determining model performance. This is clearly a major consideration in evaluating any model, so an understanding of general validation techniques is essential.

Test Population
The evaluation of any model should include an investigation of the population used to derive the model (training-set) and the population used to test the model (test-set). In some studies, the training-set and test-set populations are the same, and the validation process is termed an "intrinsic review." There are serious deficiencies with this type of analysis because the model would obviously be expected to perform well when tested against the same population used to create the model. A more rigorous assessment is obtained from the "training-set/test-set" approach in which the model is derived from one population and then tested against another entirely different group of patients. This approach is currently the accepted standard for model validation.

Predicted Versus Observed Results
The most meaningful way to assess performance is to make a direct comparison between *predicted* and *observed* results. This can be done in several ways. Initially all patient records in the test-set population are run through the model to calculate the predicted mortality for each patient. The average of these predicted probabilities represents the predicted mortality for the

COLOR PLATE I

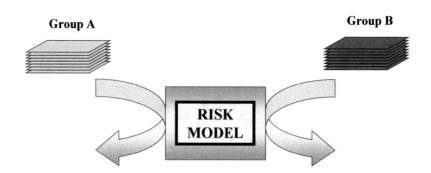

Group A

Group B

RISK MODEL

Predicted Risk - Group A

Patient #287	1%
Patient #46	1.5%
Patient #7833	1.6 %

Predicted Risk - Group B

Patient #459	0.7%
Patient #5654	1.1%
Patient #843	2.6 %

FIGURE 1.

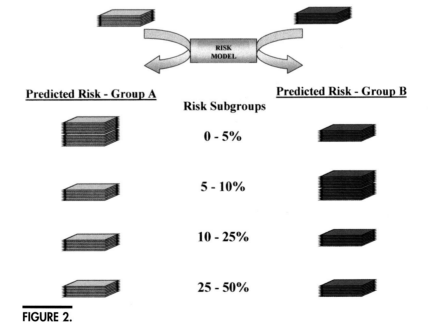

RISK MODEL

Predicted Risk - Group A

Risk Subgroups

Predicted Risk - Group B

0 - 5%

5 - 10%

10 - 25%

25 - 50%

FIGURE 2.

Risk Factors

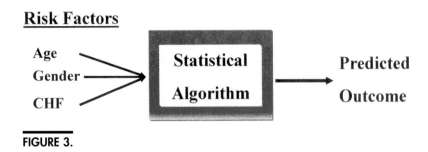

Age
Gender
CHF

Statistical Algorithm

Predicted Outcome

FIGURE 3.

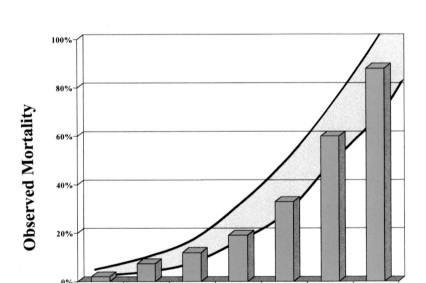

FIGURE 4.

entire test-set. The observed (actual) mortality of the test-set is then compared with the predicted mortality to see whether a statistically significant difference exists. A more challenging test involves dividing the test-set into subgroups and then comparing predicted results with observed results for each subgroup. This type of analysis allows one to assess model performance in specific parts of the risk spectrum (Fig 4; see color plate II). The subgroups typically are selected to represent clinically important risk categories, but the exact cutoff points are not well defined and are subject to individual preference. Furthermore, cutoff points can be arbitrarily selected to obscure deficiencies in the model. To obviate this unfortunate circumstance, one may create subgroups having equal numbers of patients or subgroups having equal numbers of deaths, thereby removing any subjectivity from the process. The observed mortality in these objective subgroups is then statistically compared with the predicted mortality in the group.

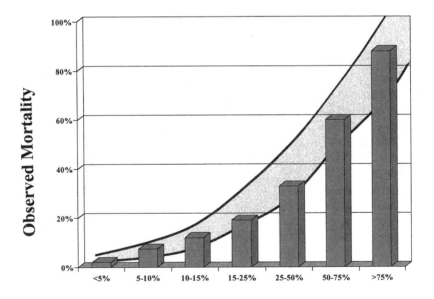

Predicted Mortality

FIGURE 4.
Predicted versus observed mortality. The *curved lines* represent the range of the respective risk categories specified on the abscissa. The *bars* denote the observed (actual) mortality for each risk category. In this example, there is good agreement between predicted and observed results.

Statistical Indices

Several statistical methods are used to provide information about model performance. In some cases, the statistical variance R^2 is calculated as a measure of overall model performance. The Breier's score, initially used in weather forecasting, has been advocated by others and may have some practical utility in this field. For practical purposes, however, most current models are evaluated using the c-statistic and the Hosmer-Lemeshow tests.

The *c-statistic*, also called the *c-index*, is calculated from a graph in which true-positive values are plotted against false-positive values (Fig 5). Such graphs are known as receiver operator characteristic curves, and the c-statistic is simply the area under the receiver operator characteristic curve. In general, the c-index

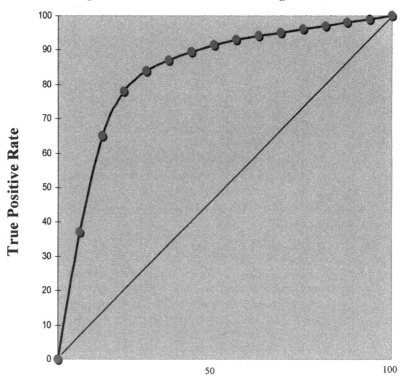

False Positive Rate

FIGURE 5.

Receiver operating characteristic curve. The *area beneath the curve* gives the c-index. The *diagonal line* represents an index that has no discrimination between outcomes.

determines the ability of the model to discriminate between possible outcomes, with higher values more desirable. As a rough estimate, a c-index greater than 0.75 would be expected in models that perform well. It is distinctly uncommon to find c-index values higher than 0.85, even in the best models.

The *Hosmer-Lemeshow test* provides an index of model calibration, which refers to the performance of the model across the entire risk spectrum. It is specified as a number less than 1.0, with higher values indicating better model calibration. If the model performs well in some areas of the risk spectrum but poorly in others, the Hosmer-Lemeshow (H-L) index will be low. This goodness-of-fit index, however, is very sensitive to the size of the patient population, thereby making interpretation difficult. In spite of this, the H-L index continues to be used frequently, so an understanding of the concept is useful. At best, the H-L index should be interpreted with caution. An analysis of predicted versus observed results across the risk spectrum is probably more useful.

THE SOCIETY OF THORACIC SURGEONS NATIONAL DATABASE

With this background, one may fully appreciate the contribution of the STS Database to our specialty. The STS Database contains records of more than 1 million patients, thereby making it the largest cardiac surgery database in the world. The database has come to be regarded as a valuable resource to cardiac surgeons, and its risk assessment algorithms are generally accepted as standard benchmarks in coronary bypass surgery.

EVOLUTION OF THE STS DATABASE

In the early 1980s, coronary bypass surgery was enjoying a "golden period" characterized by operative mortality rates of 1% to 2%. Some 5 or 6 years later, however, the landscape had dramatically changed. Urgent and emergent operations were on the increase, "redo" procedures became common, and percutaneous revascularization absorbed low-risk patients from the surgery pool. The operative mortality predictably increased to 5% to 6%. More patients were leaving the hospital alive and well, but a significant number of patients that previously would have died on the medicine ward now were dying postoperatively on the surgical service.

This increase in operative mortality was understood by cardiovascular specialists, but others were unaware of the changes that had produced these higher mortality rates. Quite appropriately, hospital administrators began to ask surgeons to justify the observed increase in CABG mortality. This usually necessitated a lengthy and often expensive chart review to document the risk factors of patients undergoing CABG. Even with this information, it proved difficult to *objectively* determine the impact of the more compelling risk factors. Although it could be shown that patients were certainly at higher risk, it was impossible to show that this higher risk would necessarily bring about the observed increase in operative mortality.

It soon became apparent that the simple collection of raw data was inadequate. To properly analyze these new patient risk factors required risk models that could generate a predicted operative mortality based on the results of an accepted standard of care.[2,3] Unfortunately, this type of analysis was unavailable to the great majority of surgical groups.

To compound these issues, in 1986 the Health Care Financing Administration released raw CABG operative mortality data into the public domain. This information soon found its way into the press, and suddenly surgeons found the operative results of their hospital in the newspaper. This was clearly an injustice to surgeons, hospitals, and patients alike, but the ill-advised precedent had been set.

Recognizing the need for an objective national standard, The Society of Thoracic Surgeons responded by appointing a formal committee to develop a national cardiac surgery database. This committee, under the leadership of Dr Richard E. Clark, was charged with the responsibility to gather and to analyze patient data in a manner that would establish a national standard of care in cardiac surgery.

Most surgeons recognized the need for this database and voluntarily participated. After the first major data harvest, Bayesian risk models of CABG operative mortality were developed, validated, and incorporated into the database software. As participation in the STS Database grew, the models shifted away from Bayesian methods in favor of the more traditional logistic regression models. Several detailed reviews of the modeling process were obtained from nationally recognized consultants to ensure rigorous adherence to the highest scientific standards.

The standard software package contains the risk algorithm for CABG operative mortality. In recent years, the algorithm has been revised with the annual data harvest, and the new risk model has then been provided to subscribers for local use.

Presently, the STS Database enrollment covers more than 80% of cardiac surgery centers in this country, and the number of registered patients is greater than 1 million. There is general, if not universal agreement that the accumulated information represents a national standard of care.

APPLICATIONS OF THE STS DATABASE
Individual Risk Assessment
Risk factors for an individual patient can be entered into the software to generate a predicted operative mortality associated with CABG. It is important to note that the model does not predict "survival" or "death" but rather provides an estimate of the *probability* of operative death based on the accumulated experience contained in this national registry. The predicted probability obtained from this model essentially tells the surgeon how a patient with this degree of comorbidity would be expected to fare based on a national standard of care.

This has obvious applications in patient counseling and medical decision-making. It should be emphasized, however, that the predicted mortality does not *dictate* patient management. These results should be regarded as a single piece to the puzzle and interpreted in concert with the other, more traditional aspects of patient care.

Quality Improvement
The STS risk models can be used as quality improvement tools using the techniques described in The Big Picture section above. There is no need for direct hospital-to-hospital comparisons, because the model itself represents the standard against which results are to be compared. Certainly such comparisons can be made, however, by providing a common yardstick to measure each institution.

In the STS system, user institutions are provided periodic reports in which their risk-adjusted results are compared with the national average experience. Options exist for individual groups to carry out a local analysis of the operative results for individual surgeons. If users find that their results are comparable to those of the STS Database, then one could logically conclude that their surgical care is in keeping with an accepted standard. On the other hand, if the results significantly deviate from those of the database, a closer inspection seems warranted. It is important to note that being identified as an "outlier" is not a form of condemnation. The STS Database Committee does not consider such "outlier" status as a marker of substandard care, but it does imply that a local examination of operative results may be in order.

Managed Care Responses
In recent years, countless practices have received requests—or demands—from managed care groups seeking detailed information on operative results. For example, in the mid-1990s, many cardiac surgery groups were notified by U.S. Healthcare that con-

tinued membership in their group would be predicated on a concise and accurate reporting system, as well as a risk assessment protocol to evaluate operative results. The STS Database was able to provide an ideal solution to these requirements, thereby allowing participating institutions to comply with the reporting mandate without expensive and time-intensive chart reviews or statistical consultations. In an excellent recent publication,[12] Dr Richard Clark provides several vignettes that illustrate this concept clearly. It appears that managed care organizations have recognized the importance of risk stratification and will often insist on this type of analysis as a condition for enrollment.

State Regulatory Requirements

Several state regulatory agencies have arbitrarily mandated that cardiac surgery centers submit morbidity and mortality data. In many instances it is all too apparent that the agencies have little expertise in this complex field, and the administrative burdens placed on the surgeon have been both oppressive and nonproductive. Fortunately, some states have come to recognize the comprehensive nature of the STS Database and have allowed centers to provide patient information in the standard STS format. Other state agencies have shown more interest in justifying their own existence and have insisted on their own unique reporting format along with risk algorithms designed by individuals with minimal understanding of cardiac surgery. The STS Database Committee has recognized that this is likely to be a recurring phenomenon and, in concert with the STS Database Liaison Committee, has developed a formal program to assist states facing regulatory mandates of this sort. Ideally, the STS and the cooperating state surgery centers will present a unified front encouraging state regulatory agencies to follow a more rational approach in which cardiac surgery results will be monitored using STS Database information.

Surgical Research

Risk models may be used as powerful research tools, particularly in the field of "single-factor analysis." In this type of study, the goal is to determine the influence of a single factor on operative outcome. The study group is divided into one population in which the factor is present and another in which it is absent. Models are used to account for the impact of all significant risk factors to create risk-matched subgroups in each of the two populations. These matched subgroups will then differ only in the presence or absence of the factor being investigated, so any significant difference in outcome will necessarily be attributed to the influence of that factor.

The STS Database has been carefully studied to identify clinically useful information of importance in cardiac surgery. To date, all published studies have dealt exclusively with coronary bypass surgery. Single-factor analysis has been used in conjunction with the STS risk models to isolate the influence of internal mammary artery grafts[13] and to investigate the impact of gender[14] on CABG outcome. In each of these studies, the protocol described above was used to definitively isolate the investigated factor to determine its influence on operative mortality. Studies are presently underway to determine the impact of retrograde cardioplegia and research proposals have been submitted to examine the role of race on CABG mortality.

DATABASE CONSIDERATIONS

Probably the most important element of any risk stratification program is the database that contains the patient risk factors and associated outcomes.[8] Informed use of risk assessment models requires some basic knowledge of the database used to develop these tools.

NATURE OF PARTICIPATION

Virtually all current risk models are generated from patient information housed in a database. These databases may be generated from voluntary contributions, as with the STS Database, or they may be associated with mandated, involuntary submission of data as seen in the New York State effort[1] or the Veterans Administration Cardiac Surgery Risk Assessment Program.[15] The strict regulatory control of the involuntary databases may be unsavory, but it does serve to ensure very good data quality and compliance. Such authority to regulate participant input is not present in the voluntary database, thereby raising questions about the completeness and consistency of the associated data. The STS Database has appointed an audit subcommittee to specifically address such concerns. Both clinical input and statistical analysis are used to screen data to ensure the highest possible quality. When evaluating a database and its associated risk model, the participatory nature should be noted and the provisions to ensure data quality should be scrutinized.

DEFINITIONS

Unfortunately, there are few instances in which a model developed from one population can be used to evaluate patients from another population. The major impediment is the inconsistency in definitions used in each population. One group, for example, may define "diabetes" as the need for insulin therapy, whereas another may consider diet or any other form of diabetic control to constitute diabetes. The precise definition of "unstable angina" is variable, but this parameter often appears as a risk factor in many models. Inconsistencies like these *absolutely preclude* a simple exchange of models from different populations.

GAMING

As mentioned above, risk-adjusted mortality has come to be an essential element in the assessment of operative results. In general, of course, risk models will predict higher operative mortality for those patients having more compelling risk factors. Recognition of this has led to the unfortunate temptation to exaggerate the severity of preoperative risk factors. This "gaming" of the system has the potential to contaminate the entire database by distorting the statistical link between important risk factors and the associated outcome. The involuntary databases neutralize this tendency by conducting on-site audits to ensure that database coding is consistent with the documented status of the patient. With voluntary databases, the issue is more challenging. The STS Database conducts an analysis of the reporting patterns of each participant for comparison with national norms. Outliers are provided information regarding their status and are encouraged to locally examine their policies.

GEOGRAPHIC SCOPE: REGIONAL VERSUS NATIONAL MODELS

The implicit assumption of a national database is that a national standard of care in cardiac surgery exists. Although this assumption is most likely true, it is conceivable that regional differences and local referral patterns could be too diverse to permit reliable comparisons with an aggregate national standard. This may be a consideration for practices that are heavily specialized in a particular area of cardiac surgery, but the nature of risk adjustment will make this a moot point for the great majority.

FUTURE DIRECTION

Future efforts will focus on the development of risk models to predict serious operative morbidity as well as mortality. Models will also be derived to predict outcomes associated with valve operations and congenital cardiac surgical procedures. Of particular interest is the standardized set of definitions being developed by a joint effort of the American College of Cardiology and The Society of Thoracic Surgeons. This set of definitions will create a vital common ground for the profession and will allow more facile communication between databases of each organization. In addition, compliance with this set of standardized definitions will allow free exchange of risk models between various populations. Clearly, large multi-institutional databases and their associated risk assessment modules serve as an extraordinarily valuable resource that will continue to have considerable impact on the practice of cardiothoracic surgery.

REFERENCES

1. Hannan EL, Kilburn H Jr, O'Donnell JF, et al: Adult open heart surgery in New York State: An analysis of risk factors and hospital mortality rates. *JAMA* 264:2768-2772, 1990.
2. Kouchoukos NT, Ebert PA, Grover FL, et al: Report of the ad hoc committee on risk factors for coronary artery bypass surgery. *Ann Thorac Surg* 45:348-349, 1988.
3. Edwards FH, Clark RE, Schwartz M: Coronary artery bypass grafting: The Society of Thoracic Surgeons National Database experience. *Ann Thorac Surg* 57:12-19, 1994.
4. Edwards FH, Grover FL, Shroyer AL, et al: The Society of Thoracic Surgeons National Cardiac Surgery Database: Current risk assessment. *Ann Thorac Surg* 63:903-908, 1997.
5. Shroyer AL, Grover FL, Edwards FH: 1995 Coronary artery bypass risk model: The Society of Thoracic Surgeons Adult Cardiac National Database. *Ann Thorac Surg* 65:879-884, 1998.
6. Edwards FH, Clark RE, Schwartz M: Practical considerations in the management of large multi-institutional databases. *Ann Thorac Surg* 58:1841-1844, 1994.
7. Parsonnet V, Dean D, Bernstein AD: A method of uniform stratification of risk for evaluating the results of surgery in acquired adult heart disease. *Circulation* 79:I3-I12, 1989.
8. Ferraris V: Risk stratification and comorbidity, in Edmunds LH (ed): *Cardiac Surgery in the Adult*. New York, McGraw-Hill, 1997, pp 165-190.
9. Marshall G, Shroyer ALW, Grover FL, et al: Bayesian-logit model for risk assessment in coronary artery bypass grafting. *Ann Thorac Surg* 57:1492-1500, 1994.
10. Daley J: Criteria by which to evaluate risk-adjusted outcomes programs in cardiac surgery. *Ann Thorac Surg* 58:1827-1835, 1994.
11. Edwards FH, Graeber GM: The theorem of Bayes as a clinical research tool. *Surg Gynecol Obstet* 165:127-129, 1987.

12. Clark RE: The STS Cardiac Surgery National Database: An update. *Ann Thorac Surg* 59:1376-1381, 1995.
13. Edwards FH, Clark RE, Schwartz M: The impact of internal mammary artery conduits on operative mortality in coronary revascularization. *Ann Thorac Surg* 57:27-32, 1994.
14. Edwards FH, Carey JS, Grover FL, et al: The impact of gender on coronary bypass operative mortality. *Ann Thorac Surg* 66:125-131, 1998.
15. Hammermeister KE, Johnson R, Marshall G, et al: Continuous assessment and improvement in quality of care: A model from the Department of Veterans Affairs Cardiac Surgery. *Ann Surg* 219:281-290, 1994.

CHAPTER 6

The Electrophysiologist and the Cardiac Surgeon

Louis E. Samuels, MD
Assistant Professor of Cardiothoracic Surgery, MCP Hahnemann
University; Director of Clinical Research, Hahnemann University
Hospital, Philadelphia, Pennsylvania

Fania L. Samuels, MD
Clinical Assistant Professor of Medicine, Division of Cardiology, MCP
Hahnemann University; Staff, Department of Electrophysiology,
Hahnemann University Hospital, Philadelphia, Pennsylvania

Historically, the identification and treatment of cardiac arrhythmias were shared by physician and surgeon alike. During the early years of surgical management for congenital heart disease, arrhythmia and heart block were among the leading causes of perioperative death. With the clinical introduction of cardiac defibrillation in the 1940s and direct myocardial pacing in the 1950s, mortality rates dropped considerably. In the past 50 years, refinements in arrhythmia determination and therapy have resulted in an "industrialized revolution" in antiarrhythmic technology. In the wake of this technological explosion, new and improved device designs and components have rapidly and regularly appeared on the American and European markets. Simultaneously, innovative surgical techniques and procedures have been designed both to treat and prevent atrial and ventricular arrhythmias. The purpose of this chapter is to update the cardiac surgeon in the evolving field of electrophysiology as it pertains to cardiac surgery. No attempt is made to review the literature or address the multitude of antiarrhythmic pharmacotherapeutic agents. Rather, useful information and guidelines are presented, with emphasis on common practices used today and new innovations for the future.

HISTORICAL BACKGROUND

The 1940s and 1950s were pioneering times for cardiothoracic surgeons. Created in 1948, the American Board of Thoracic Surgery was founded, recognizing the field as a specialized area of surgery. Although direct coronary arterial revascularization was not to appear for another two decades, surgical intervention for congenital heart disease and cardiac valvular disease was initiated and promoted. In this setting, the recognition and appreciation of arrhythmias was apparent. Whether preoperative, perioperative, or postoperative, cardiac arrhythmias and heart block were leading causes of death in these populations. Indeed, until isoproterenol was used, surgical heart block was uniformly fatal.

Beginning in 1947, Beck et al[1] were the first to use internal defibrillation in the clinical setting. Nearly 10 years later, Zoll et al[2] performed the first transthoracic direct current defibrillation. In the same year, Brockman et al[3] were the first to use a myocardial pacing electrode to manage postoperative heart block after repair of a congenital ventricular septal defect. During the 1960s, several investigators described advances in pacemaker design and use.[4-6] The majority of these investigators were surgeons because the initial pacemakers were placed directly on the epicardium of the heart. In the 1970s, experimental work on termination of ventricular fibrillation (VF) with an automatic and implantable defibrillator was conducted.[7,8] In 1980, Mirowski et al[9] were the first to report the clinical use of an implantable cardiac defibrillator. Between 1980 and the present, pacemaker and defibrillator design and capability have progressed to unimaginable levels. Pacemakers as small as a half dollar with variable rate responsive features and defibrillators smaller than a pack of cigarettes with antitachycardia pacing functions and dual-chamber pacing capabilities were among the advances seen in this field. As a result of the reduction in generator size, coupled with transvenous lead deployment, the cardiothoracic surgeon has been displaced by the cardiologist in primary implantation procedures. Electrophysiologists, a special breed of cardiologist requiring specific board certification, are now occupying the domain of what was once a surgical field. Indeed, ablative procedures, once an operation of considerable magnitude performed by a selective number of cardiothoracic surgeons, have been transformed into a transvenous approach using radiofrequency performed in the laboratory by cardiologists.

Despite the evolution of the field of electrophysiology away from cardiothoracic surgeons, our knowledge of and expertise in dealing with the cardiac conduction system, as well as our knowledge of the surgical anatomy of the heart, require us to participate in arrhythmia therapy. Among our areas of involvement today include complex implants or explants of devices, management of complications from device deployment or ablative therapy, device creation and testing in surgical patients, and surgical management of arrhythmia in the setting of failed medical therapy (eg, intractable ventricular and supraventricular tachycardia). In the following sections, emphasis is placed on the surgical participation within the field of electrophysiology.

PACEMAKERS

The history of cardiac pacemakers is rich with creative and innovative designs and capabilities. In general, the trend has been toward a smaller and more sophisticated model that could be easily deployed. Hence, the infraclavicular subcutaneous generator with transvenous atrioventricular (AV) leads is now the standard device used. However, a discussion of epicardial as well as endocardial systems is necessary, because both remain in use today.

EPICARDIAL
Temporary

Epicardial pacemaker systems must be categorized into those for temporary use and those for permanent use. Temporary epicardial pacemakers are among the most commonly used devices in cardiac surgery. Although the leads and generators have undergone some refinement over the decades, little has changed in their design and function. Basically, a simple wire lead is attached to the epicardial surface of the atrium or ventricle, brought through the skin, and attached to an external pulse generator. The ability to pace the atria and ventricles in a synchronous or asynchronous fashion is standard for today's generators. More sophisticated generators are available but are rarely necessary. In the author's (LES) opinion, the older model generator is more "user friendly" than is the newer one because pacemaker parameters can be simply changed by turning a dial instead of a push-button digital display programmer, and a "pause button" is available to easily evaluate underlying rhythms without losing the memory of the previous setting. Overall, regardless of the system, the equipment is simple, inexpensive, and reliable. There are few complications.

Recently, several technical items have been recognized by ourselves and others. In a study at our institution, atrial lead placement within the pursestring of the atrial appendage—a practice borne out of convenience—was associated with suboptimal pacing thresholds.[10] On the first postoperative day, only 58% of purse-string atrial wires captured; on the second postoperative day, only 40% captured. Furthermore, the mean threshold for atrial capture was higher in the pursestring group than in the non-pursestring group (Table 1). Thus, placing a pacing electrode within crushed atrial tissue resulted in suboptimal pacing. Based on this experience, this practice has been abandoned. Instead, the leads are placed outside the pursestring on the body of the atrium.

Additional use of the atrial wires has been seen in rhythm identi-fication and treatment. Atrial flutter, for example, can be easily iden-tified by performing atrial electrograms at the bedside. The atrial leads are attached to the clips of the skin leads electrocardiography. The electrical impulse of the atrium is transmitted across the atrial electrode and registered on the electrocardiography screen, thereby demonstrating an atrial electrogram. Based on the rate and regularity of the atrial electrogram, rhythm identification can be achieved. Furthermore, overdrive pacing can be performed through the inter-nal leads for successful cardioversion. At the bedside, the atrial wires

---

TABLE 1.

Mean Threshold, Number of Captures, and Changes in Mean Threshold

	Appendage	**Body**
Mean threshold (mA) on:		
Op day	5.98 (2-11)	4.96 (2-10)
POD 1	7.50 (3-11)	6.67 (3-15)
POD 2	8.59 (4-13)	6.80 (3-16)
Number (%) of noncaptures on:		
Op day	2 (3.6%)	0 (0%)
POD 1	23 (41.8%)	0 (0%)
POD 2	33 (60.0%)	5 (9.1%)
Change in mean threshold (mA) from:		
Op day to POD 1	(+) 1.52	(+) 1.71
Op day to POD 2	(+) 2.61	(+) 1.84
POD 1 to POD 2	(+) 1.09	(+) 0.13

Abbreviations: Op, operative; *POD,* postoperative day.
(Courtesy of Samuels LE, Samuels FL, Kaufman MS, et al: Temporary epicardial atrial pacing electrodes: Duration of effectiveness based on position. *Am J Med Sci* 315:248-250, 1998.)

are attached to a special atrial pacing pulse generator capable of providing up to 1200 stimuli per minute. Atrial stimulation is initiated and increased in a gradual fashion. Once atrial capture is confirmed, the rate is increased to a level above the flutter rate (300-400 beats/min). Pacing is performed for a short interval (5-10 seconds), and then the rate is reduced until the patient's sinus rhythm is reestablished. The results of this procedure are variable, and multiple attempts may be necessary before successful cardioversion is accomplished. Additional pharmacotherapy is often necessary (eg, β-blocker or calcium channel blocker), and reduction or elimination of inotropic agents is desirable. The advantages of atrial flutter cardioversion with overdrive atrial pacing are several: it can be done at the bedside, it is simple to perform, it is noninvasive, and it is relatively effective.

In addition to the above, the internal temporary epicardial atrial wires can be used for atrial fibrillation (AF) prevention and treatment. Placement of right atrial leads in two locations—high near the sinoatrial node and low near the coronary sinus—has been used

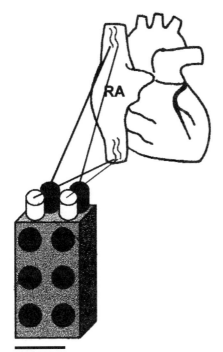

FIGURE 1.
Configuration of temporary atrial electrodes for dual-site atrial pacing. *Abbreviation: RA,* right atrium.

for dual-site atrial pacing for AF prevention (Fig 1).[11] Post-operatively, the unipolar leads are connected as follows: the superior lead to the atrial channel of the external pacemaker and the inferior lead to the ventricular channel. The leads are grounded to external, low-impedance, skin electrodes (stick-on). The shortest possible delay (0-6 msec) between the two leads is programmed. The atrial pacing is set at 10 to 15 beats/min greater than the underlying rate to override normal sinus rhythm. Dual-site atrial pacing is continued for 3 postoperative days. On the fourth postoperative day, the atrial pacing is gradually weaned off over 1 to 2 hours. The preliminary results at our institution indicate a modest reduction in AF compared with age-, sex-, and procedure-matched counterparts. The earlier recovery of excitability with elimination of a potential zone of slow conduction with this pacing mode could be the mechanism of AF prevention.[12] Finally, the use of these electrodes for internal atrial defibrillation will be discussed in a later section.

In summary, temporary epicardial pacing electrodes and generators remain an important and common adjunct to the cardiac surgeon. Their use has evolved beyond pacemaking to include arrhythmia identification, prevention, and treatment.

Permanent

Permanent epicardial pacemaker leads are available as screw-in (active fixation) or tined types (passive fixation). Although permanent epicardial pacemakers were used commonly in the past, they are rarely used today. The indication for their application is the inability to place an endovascular lead. This situation may arise in patients with congenital or acquired stenosis of the central veins, or the presence of other material in the central venous system (eg, dialysis catheters, Hickmann catheters), making transvenous access unobtainable or ill-advised. A recent example at our institution of a condition for preferred epicardial approach was a patient with superior vena cava (SVC) syndrome from pre-existing central venous leads.[13] After surgical correction of the stenotic SVC, permanent tined-type electrodes were placed on the right atrium and right ventricle. A subcostal generator was implanted within the subcutaneous tissue. Finally, on sternal closure, a GoreTex (W.L. Gore and Associates, Inc., Flagstaff, Ariz) pericardial patch was placed in the event of a future sternotomy. Avoidance of the SVC repair, provision for long-term pacing capability, and application of a pericardial barrier for safe sternal reentry in the future were the principles of the procedure performed in this case and others requiring permanent epicardial pacemakers.

ENDOCARDIAL

Endocardial, endovascular, or transvenous leads are the most common types used for permanent pacemaker use. Screw-in and tined types are available, with specific reasons to use one or the other. In general, screw-in leads are easier to implant, but there is a greater risk of perforation. The tined leads are reported to have better long-term pacing thresholds but are difficult to use in the atrial position of patients after open-heart surgery in which the appendage was ligated. In the coauthor's (FLS) opinion, large dilated or hypertrophic hearts are better served with screw-in leads; tined leads are safer in small, older hearts. In general, the choice of lead is at the implanter's discretion.

From the surgical perspective, placement of the leads and creation of the generator pocket has been simplified and standardized to the point that most systems are deployed by nonsurgeons. Occasionally, surgeons are consulted for difficult lead placement, alternative sites for generator location, complications from device placement, and management of infected systems.

An interesting procedure now performed with some regularity is percutaneous lead extraction. The indications and technique of lead extraction have been well described by Kantharia and Kutalek.[14] At our institution, lead extraction has been performed in more than 400 patients with excellent results (98% success rate). Although surgical standby was routinely provided during the initial experience, the technique is currently performed by electrophysiologists in their procedure room. Despite the potential for serious complications, the actual occurrence is relatively rare (0.7%). Surgical intervention has been used for cardiac tamponade in only two cases.

DEFIBRILLATORS

Defibrillators were developed to address a population of patients who died of sudden cardiac death (SCD) secondary to ventricular dysrhythmia. In the United States alone, 400,000 individuals die of SCD annually. Although the etiology of SCD is multifactorial, the final common pathway appears to be a ventricular dysrhythmia. The rhythm may begin as ventricular tachycardia (VT) initially, disorganize into VF, and ultimately degenerate into asystole. Hence, the design of defibrillators has evolved from a device that recognizes the dysrhythmia and provides an appropriate shock, to a system that can provide antitachycardia and dual-chamber pacing if asystole, bradycardia, or heart block accompanies the condition.

EPICARDIAL

The early-generation defibrillators were placed in the operating room under direct vision. Large patches were positioned on the anterior and posterior aspects of the heart. These patches were connected by a lead to a large generator that was positioned in the subcostal region under the rectus abdominis muscle or fascia. The patches and generators were sometimes placed at the time of corrective cardiac surgery (eg, coronary artery bypass graft) and sometimes as an isolated procedure. When performed as an isolated procedure, the choice of sternotomy, thoracotomy, or subxiphoid window was left to the surgeon's discretion. Irrespective of the approach at insertion, removal can be hazardous. Whether removal is performed for infection or as part of another procedure, the patches can be densely adherent to the heart. Although the anterior patch may be removed without too much difficulty, removal of the posterior patch can be life-threatening.[15] Therefore, unless the patches are grossly infected or unless removal is vital to the operation being performed, a difficult patch removal should be abandoned. Fortunately, the technology of implantable defibrillators has progressed toward smaller patches and generators. Simultaneously, technology evolved to permit transvenous electrodes. A short period existed in which there was overlap with epicardial patches and transvenous electrodes. With further refinement in technology, the entire system is now placed in an endovascular manner with an infraclavicular generator implant.

ENDOCARDIAL

The endocardial (or endovascular) system is the current technology that is in use today. Whereas two transvenous leads were required a short time ago—one positioned in the SVC and the other in the right ventricle—at present, both sensing and defibrillating coils are incorporated into a single lead. This electrode is attached to a generator that has been reduced in size to permit subpectoral, and most recently, subcutaneous implantation. The reduction in size of the generator, coupled with the simplicity of lead insertion, has permitted electrophysiologists to place devices in their laboratory without surgical assistance. Except for complex or difficult implants, the majority of defibrillators are placed by cardiologists.

One important area of surgical involvement includes removal of infected hardware. In a study at our institution, the management of infected defibrillators is subject to significant morbidity and mortality.[16] As a general rule, infected units should be completely removed. As opposed to the hazards of removing epicardial defibrillating patches, removal of transvenous systems is much safer. In addition to removing the hardware, antibiotics should be continued until all evidence of active or ongoing infection is eliminated. New equipment should be replaced in an area remote from the infected site. Although leaving the "clean" electrode and removing and replacing the "dirty" generator has been done, this practice is not advised. Persistent infection or reappearance of smoldering infection will occur in a subset of patients, making management more complex and costly.

ABLATIVE THERAPY FOR VENTRICULAR TACHYARRHYTHMIAS
SURGICAL

The possibility of surgical ablation of VT was realized when Couch[17] made the association of cardiac aneurysm with VT. The arrhythmia was eradicated by excision of the aneurysm. The curative surgical approach to ventricular tachyarrhythmia

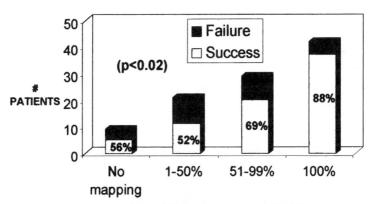

FIGURE 2.
Influence of mapping on surgical outcome for ventricular tachycardia (*VT*). (Courtesy of Josephson ME: Surgical and nonsurgical ablation in the therapy of arrhythmias, in Josephson ME [ed]: *Clinical Cardiac Electrophysiology Techniques and Interpretations,* ed 2. Philadelphia, Lea & Febiger, 1993, p 803.)

depends on specific mapping of the suspected arrhythmogenic area. Although "blind" endocardial resection has been done with variable success, the results are clearly superior with electrophysiologic mapping (Fig 2).[18] The reasons for the superior results observed with mapping are as follows: (1) 15% of tachycardias arise outside regions of visible scar or abnormal electrograms, (2) visible landmarks of the entire arrhythmogenic substrate are not distinct and well defined in the setting of recent myocardial infarction, and (3) tachycardias may arise in deeper areas of the myocardium that would not be normally addressed by routine non–map-guided procedures. The technique and outcomes of surgical ablative therapy for VT have been well documented by Harken[19] and others. Guidelines regarding the choice of endocardial resection versus implantable cardiac defibrillator (ICD) implantation have been suggested by Cleveland and Harken.[20] The algorithm they present serves as a useful guide for determining the appropriate mode of therapy (Fig 3). Despite the excellent success at eradicating VT with endocardial resection,

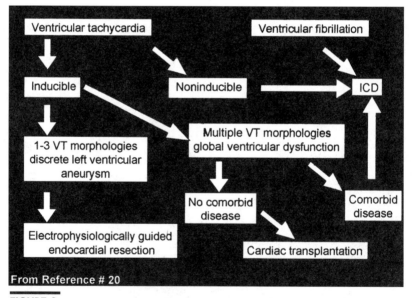

From Reference # 20

FIGURE 3.
Factors influencing surgical therapy versus implantable cardiac defibrillator *(ICD)* therapy for ventricular tachycardia *(VT)*. Therapeutic algorithm is shown. (Courtesy of Cleveland JC Jr, Harken AH: Rational strategies in the surgical therapy of malignant ventricular tachyarrhythmias, in *Mastery of Cardiothoracic Surgery.* Philadelphia, Lippincott-Raven, 1998, p 545.)

the increased perioperative mortality and morbidity make this procedure undesirable by some surgeons and cardiologists. Concomitantly, the less-invasive advantage of ICDs and percutaneous ablative therapy make these procedures attractive. The choice of therapy depends on a joint decision of surgeon and electrophysiologist and must be individualized for each patient.

INTERVENTIONAL

Although the initial experience with catheter ablation of VT had been disappointing, more recent reports have demonstrated improved results.[21,22] The ablative techniques that are under experimental investigation or are being used clinically include (1) electrical fulguration, (2) nonarcing electrical shocks, (3) laser vaporization (argon) or photocoagulation (Nd:YAG), (4) chemical destruction, (5) cryothermal ablation, and (6) radiofrequency thermal injury and desiccation. New forms of energy, such as microwaves, are currently being investigated. It is beyond the scope and purpose of this chapter to discuss the characteristics of each method. Interested readers are referred to specific electrophysiology textbooks and journals.

The important points regarding interventional management of VT are that it is being done with increasing frequency, requires sophisticated mapping, provides successful ablation in certain subsets of VT, and is less risky than endocardial resection. The limitations of this technique are the inability to map and ablate the specific arrhythmia site, the inability to access the specific arrhythmia site, and recurrence of the arrhythmia after "successful" ablation. In general, surgical involvement for interventional ablative therapy is necessary only for procedure-related complications, venous access difficulty, and failure of therapy.

ABLATIVE THERAPY FOR SUPRAVENTRICULAR TACHYARRHYTHMIAS
SURGICAL

The development of surgical techniques to cure supraventricular arrhythmias began with the first successful electrophysiologically directed cure of the Wolff-Parkinson-White syndrome by Sealy et al[23] in 1968. This event initiated the development and continued refinement of surgical techniques to manage other supraventricular disorders, including AV nodal reentrant tachycardia, atrial tachycardias, and atrial flutter and fibrillation.[24-27] Although it is beyond the scope of this chapter to review the surgical techniques of these procedures, it is worth commenting on the indications and results of one of the more well-known operations, the Maze procedure.

Beginning with experimental studies in the 1970s, a series of operations were devised by Cox and others to treat AF. Based on left atrial isolation and the corridor procedure introduced in the 1980s, creation of a technique that would achieve interruption of all potential reentrant circuits was devised and modified into what is now referred to as the Maze III. In essence, atrial incisions are appropriately placed to interrupt the conduction routes of the most common reentrant circuits while still permitting conduction of the sinus impulse to the AV node and to all portions of the right and left atrial myocardium to obtain synchronous contraction of both atria and a normal PR interval. The modifications were made to simplify the procedure, improve the synchrony of atrial contraction, and avoid blunting the normal sinus tachycardia response to exercise. The indications for the Maze procedure include (1) failure of medical therapy as a result of symptomatic intolerance of the arrhythmia despite pharmacologic rate control, or an inability to achieve satisfactory pharmacologic rate control; (2) patient intolerance of the requisite drug therapy; or (3) the occurrence of at least one previous thromboembolic episode attributable to the dysrhythmia. The results of the Maze procedure have improved significantly with the modifications made. The long-term results demonstrate 100% cure of AF and atrial flutter (93% without drugs), 100% restoration of AV synchrony (68% without atrial pacing), and 98% right/81% left atrial transport function preservation. In short, the success of the Maze procedure has made it an attractive approach to atrial arrhythmias refractory to medical therapy or when intolerance to medical therapy occurs. According to Cox, the procedure should be given consideration during other cardiac operations when AF is present in patients for whom the atrial dysrhythmia per se was not the primary indication for surgery.

INTERVENTIONAL

The use of ablative techniques to directly manage atrial arrhythmias is fraught with the problem that there is no identifiable pathologic substrate for these arrhythmias. Thus, ablative procedures must be targeted toward the mapped arrhythmia site in the case of atrial tachycardia or the assumed critical areas involved in atrial flutter and flutter/fibrillation. As a result of this, it is not uncommon to observe a recurrent arrhythmia in what was considered an initial curative procedure.

Atrial tachycardia and atrial flutter have been the two atrial arrhythmias for which ablative therapy has been used. Atrial tachycardias can be ablated via catheter using high-energy shocks or radiofrequency. Detailed mapping is required. Poor access to the left atrium limits the performance of detailed mapping, and hence, successful catheter ablation of left atrial foci. Because the atrium is thin walled, radiofrequency ablative techniques offer the most promise for managing these arrhythmias. Catheter radiofrequency ablation has several advantages, the most important of which is the presence of the arrhythmia in the catheterization laboratory and the ability to spend time localizing it. Improvement in catheter technology and energy sources may allow more of these arrhythmias to be approached and cured than at present. Until then, the apparent high recurrence rate remains the limiting factor in atrial tachycardia.

Atrial flutter, particularly the common type, has been cured by catheter ablation. In the common type of atrial flutter, the low right atrium appears to be the culprit site. The region between the coronary sinus, inferior vena cava, and tricuspid valve appears to be a critical component of the circuit that exhibits slow conduction. Catheter-based ablation using 200 J of direct current (DC) energy to this territory has been successful. Admittedly, like atrial tachycardia, recurrence has been reported for atrial flutter ablation from 6 months to 2 years after the initial procedure.[28]

In short, management of atrial arrhythmias remains an area subject to multiple therapeutic options: pharmacologic, interventional, and surgical. The proper choice of therapy must take into consideration the advantages and disadvantages of each modality and weigh the risks and benefits accordingly.

MANAGEMENT OF PACEMAKERS AND DEFIBRILLATORS DURING OPEN-HEART SURGERY

One aspect of cardiac surgery that may be overshadowed by the magnitude of the major operative procedure is the presence and influence of a preexisting pacemaker or defibrillator. Although it may seem trivial on the surface, the presence of these devices can have profound consequences. A sudden discharge from a defibrillator while using the electrocautery may result in the production of a life-threatening arrhythmia. Similarly, use of the electrocautery in the setting of a pacemaker can reprogram the pacemaker in a suboptimal configuration, resulting in hemodynamic compromise. In fact, pacemaker function may be temporarily inhibited during electrocautery use. In a pacemaker-dependent patient, loss of function can be devastating. Finally, electrocautery can permanently alter the circuitry of either pacemaker or defibrillator, requiring removal and replacement with a new device.

The simple solution to these problems is the placement of a magnet. In the case of the defibrillator, the magnet automatically "blinds" the device, thereby preventing it from sensing and treating the electrical "noise" produced by the electrocautery. Once the magnet is removed, defibrillator function is restored. In the case of a pacemaker, the magnet causes the generator to be functional in an asynchronous fixed rate. In the operating room, the customary practice is to apply a sterile magnet over the device and fix it to the skin with suture material to prevent movement. Postoperatively, if device function is in doubt, or reprogramming is needed to adjust to postoperative conditions, device interrogation can be performed by the electrophysiologist.

RECENT DEVELOPMENTS

As we approach the next millenium, there remain several unsolved electrophysiologic problems as they relate to the field of cardiac surgery. On the atrial side, a solution to the problem of postoperative AF still eludes us. On the ventricular side, the management of refractory ventricular tachyarrhythmias remains problematic. In our field, several areas of investigation are at work to address these problems.

ATRIAL DEFIBRILLATORS

As alluded to earlier, AF is the most common arrhythmia encountered by the cardiac surgeon. Irrespective of the debate regarding its origin, AF poses several real and potential problems: decreased cardiac output, increased stroke risk, and the need for anticoagulation. Recently, atrial defibrillators have been developed and tested in the animal and human models.[29] Simultaneous development of chronic implantable devices and temporary removable systems have been studied. The chronic implantable system consists of a transvenous lead whose tip is positioned within the coronary sinus. Defibrillation occurs between two shocking coils, which are located at the right and left atrial levels (Fig 4). The early reports of this device are encouraging.[30]

The temporary removable atrial defibrillator referred to earlier is an example of using standard epicardial pacing electrodes in an innovative fashion. The same atrial leads used for postoperative pacing may be positioned at both the right and left atrium in a circular configuration for use as internal atrial defibrillators (Fig 5). In a recent report by Liebold et al,[31] atrial defibrillation was successfully and safely performed in open-heart surgical patients with a mean energy shock of 3.1 ± 1.9 J. The electrodes (TAD-Pole InControl Inc., Redmond, Wash) were stainless steel wires with a

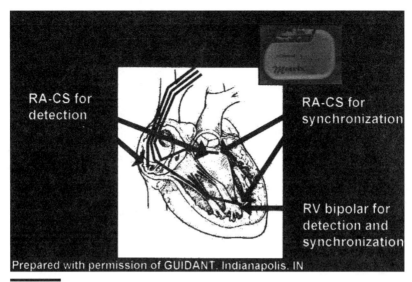

FIGURE 4.
Permanent transvenous atrial defibrillator lead configuration. *Abbreviations: RA,* right atrium; *CS,* coronary sinus; *RV,* right ventricle. (Prepared with permission of Guidant Corporation, Indianapolis, Ind.)

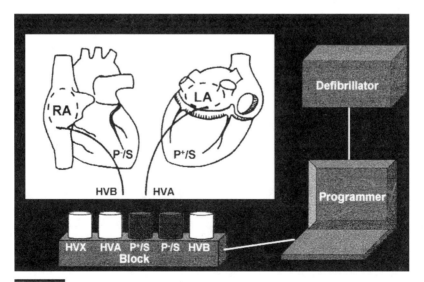

FIGURE 5.
Configuration of temporary epicardial atrial defibrillator. *Abbreviations: RA,* right atrium; *LA,* left atrium; *P/S,* pace/sense; *HVB,* high voltage cathode (-); *HVA,* high voltage anode (+); *HVX,* high voltage x-tra (+).

10-cm distal bare portion that was in direct contact with the atrial tissue. In our laboratory, we have performed similar experiments in the swine model using standard temporary epicardial pacing leads from Ethicon (Sommerville, NJ) and Medtronic (Minneapolis, Minn). Successful cardioversion was achieved with 1 J of energy.

The benefit of a temporary internal atrial defibrillator is apparent. The advantages of this system are (1) easy insertion and removal; (2) low energy requirements for internal defibrillation; (3) bedside defibrillation with minimal sedation; (4) low cost; and (5) prompt defibrillation, reducing the risk of stroke and need for anticoagulation.

In summary, atrial defibrillators, whether temporary or permanent, are fast becoming a part of cardiac surgery and electrophysiology. Until a solution is found to prevent the arrhythmia from occurring, these devices are likely to play an important role in cardiac care, postoperative or otherwise.

VENTRICULAR ASSIST DEVICES

Ventricular assist devices (VADs) were developed to assist the failing heart. Associated with the failing heart are ventricular arrhythmias, which may or may not respond to conventional antiarrhythmic therapy. In the setting of intractable, incessant ventricular tachyarrhythmia, the only remaining option is mechanical circulatory assist. In fact, this lethal condition is one of the indications for VAD support. Several authors have described successful support of patients with intractable VT on univentricular or biventricular support.[32,33] At our institution, we have had two occasions in which successful bridge to transplant was possible with VAD technology. In one patient, a Novacor left ventricular assist system (Baxter, Oakland, Calif) was placed in a patient with idiopathic dilated cardiomyopathy. Despite persistent VT, he was successfully bridged to transplant after several weeks on support. In another patient, an Abiomed Bi-VAD (Abiomed, Danvers, Mass) was placed in a woman with cardiogenic shock after a massive myocardial infarction. In the setting of VT/VF, normal hemodynamics were maintained until transplant 7 days later (Fig 6). The only problem with VAD support during VT/VF is the formation of thrombus from stagnant blood in the cardiac chambers. Despite therapeutic anticoagulation, stagnant blood has a propensity to clot. The risk of thromboembolism increases with time as long as the patient remains in this dysrhythmia. However, thromboembolism is also a problem in patients converting from VT/VF to sinus rhythm. In the new age

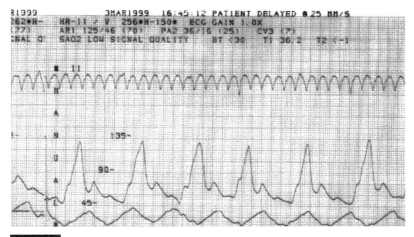

FIGURE 6.
Illustration showing circulatory support with Abiomed BVS 5000I Bi-VAD in setting of incessant ventricular tachycardia (*VT*)/ventricular fibrillation (*VF*).

of total artificial heart technology, heart failure and intractable arrhythmia may be treated with this type of total implantable circulatory assist device. Placement of an orthotopic device also eliminates the concerns about stagnant blood.

CONCLUSION

The electrophysiologist and the cardiac surgeon have had a long-term relationship that has shifted from one area of expertise to the other over the decades. Although our specialty has seen the majority of procedures removed from the operating room and into the interventional suite, we maintain a presence in complex cases and when complications occur from procedures. In addition, we are actively exploring ways in which to manage prevailing problems, particularly postoperative AF and incessant tachyarrhythmia. Our role, as cardiac surgeons, remains as investigator, applicator, and trouble-shooter.

REFERENCES

1. Beck CS, Pritchard WH, Fell HS: Ventricular fibrillation of long duration abolished by electric shock. *JAMA* 135:985-986, 1947.
2. Zoll PM, Linethal AJ, Gibson W, et al: Termination of ventricular fibrillation in man by externally applied electric shock. *N Engl J Med* 254:727-732, 1956.
3. Brockman SK, Webb RC, Bahnson HT: Monopolar ventricular stimu-

lation for the control of acute surgically produced heart block. *Surgery* 44:910-918, 1958.

4. Lillehei CW, Levy MJ, Gonnabeau RC Jr, et al: Direct wire electrical stimulation for acute postsurgical and postinfarction complete heart block. *Ann N Y Acad Sci* 3:938-949, 1964.

5. Harris PD, Singer DH, Malm JR, et al: Chronically implanted cardiac electrodes for diagnostic, therapeutic, and investigational use in man. *J Thorac Cardiovasc Surg* 54:191-198, 1967.

6. Hodam RP, Start A: Temporary postoperative epicardial pacing electrodes: Their value and management after open-heart surgery. *Ann Thorac Surg* 8:506-510, 1969.

7. Mirowski M, Mower MM, Staewen WS, et al: Standby automatic defibrillator: An approach to prevention of sudden coronary death. *Arch Intern Med* 126:158-161, 1970.

8. Shuder JC, Stoeckle H, Gold JH, et al: Experimental ventricular defibrillation with an automatic and completely implanted system. *Am Soc Artif Int Organs* 16:207-212, 1970.

9. Mirowski M, Reid PR, Mower MM, et al: Termination of malignant ventricular arrhythmias with an implanted automatic defibrillator in human beings. *N Engl J Med* 303:322-324, 1980.

10. Samuels LE, Samuels FL, Kaufman MS, et al: Temporary epicardial atrial pacing electrodes: Duration of effectiveness based on position. *Am J Med Sci* 315:248-250, 1998.

11. Solomon AJ, Verdino RJ, Katz NM: Dual site atrial pacing in cardiovascular surgical patients. *Circulation* 94:1-677S, 1996.

12. Prakash A, Saksena S, Krol RB, et al: Electrophysiology of acute prevention of atrial fibrillation and flutter with dual site right atrial pacing. *Pacing Clin Electrophysiol* 18:803, 1995.

13. Samuels LE, Nyzio J, Thomas MP: Acute superior vena cava (SVC) syndrome with SVC rupture following sinus node ablation, pacemaker placement, SVC angioplasty and stenting: Surgical and electrophysiological management [not in print].

14. Kantharia BK, Kutalek SP: Extraction of pacemaker and implantable cardioverter defibrillator leads. *Curr Opin Cardiol* 14:44-51, 1999.

15. Kassanoff AH, Levin CB, Wyndham CRC, et al: Implantable cardioverter defibrillator infection causing constrictive pericarditis. *Chest* 102:960-963, 1992.

16. Samuels LE, Samuels FL, Kaufman MS, et al: Management of infected implantable cardiac defibrillators. *Ann Thorac Surg* 64:1702-1706, 1997.

17. Couch OA: Cardiac arrhythmia with ventricular tachycardia and subsequent excision of aneurysm. *Circulation* 20:251-253, 1959.

18. Miller JM, Vassallo JA, Rosenthal ME, et al: Does ventricular tachycardia mapping influence the success of antiarrhythmic surgery? *J Am Coll Cardiol* 2:112A, 1988.

19. Harken AH: Surgical treatment of cardiac arrhythmias. *Sci Am* 269:68-74, 1993.

20. Cleveland JC Jr, Harken AH: Rational strategies in the surgical therapy of malignant ventricular tachyarrhythmias, in Kaiser LR, Kron IL, Spray TL (eds): *Mastery of Cardiothoracic Surgery.* Philadelphia, Lippincott-Raven, 1998, p 545.

21. Wilbur DJ, Baerman J, Olshansky B, et al: Adenosine-sensitive ventricular tachycardia: Clinical characteristics and response to catheter ablation. *Circulation* 87:126-134, 1993.

22. Smeets JLRM, Rodriguez LM, Metzger J, et al: Can ventricular tachycardia in the absence of structural heart disease be cured by radiofrequency catheter ablation? *Eur Heart J* 14:256S, 1993.

23. Sealy WC, Hattler BG, Blumenschein SD, et al: Surgical treatment of Wolff-Parkinson White syndrome. *Ann Thorac Surg* 8:1-11, 1969.

24. Ferguson TB Jr, Cox JL: Surgery for atrial fibrillation, in Zipes DP, Jalife J (eds): *Cardiac Electrophysiology: From Cell to Bedside.* Philadelphia, WB Saunders, 1995, pp 1563-1576.

25. Mahomed Y: Surgery for atrioventricular nodal reentrant tachycardia, in Zipes DP, Jalife J (eds): *Cardiac Electrophysiology: From Cell to Bedside.* Philadelphia, WB Saunders, 1995, pp 1577-1584.

26. Cox JL, Schuessler RB, D'Agostino, et al: The surgical treatment of atrial fibrillation: III. Development of a definitive surgical procedure. *J Thorac Cardiovasc Surg* 101:569-583, 1991.

27. Cox JL: The surgical treatment of atrial fibrillation: IV. Surgical technique. *J Thorac Cardiovasc Surg* 101:584-592, 1991.

28. Saoudi N, Atallah G, Kirkorian G, et al: Catheter ablation of the atrial myocardium in human type I atrial flutter. *Circulation* 81:762-771, 1990.

29. Hillsey RE, Wharton JM: Implantable atrial defibrillators. *J Cardiovasc Electrophysiol* 6:634-648, 1995.

30. Levy S, Ricard P, Lau C, et al: Multicenter low energy transvenous atrial defibrillation trial (XAD) results in different subsets of atrial fibrillation. *J Am Coll Cardiol* 29:750-755, 1997.

31. Liebold A, Rodig G, Bimbaum D: Performance of temporary epicardial stainless steel wire electrodes used to treat atrial fibrillation. *Pacing Clin Electrophysiol* 22:315-319, 1999.

32. Kulick DM, Bolman RM III, Salerno CT, et al: Management of recurrent ventricular tachycardia with ventricular assist device placement. *Ann Thorac Surg* 66:571-573, 1998.

33. Oz MC, Rose EA, Slater J, et al: Malignant ventricular arrhythmias are well tolerated in patients receiving long-term left ventricular assist devices. *J Am Coll Cardiol* 24:1688-1691, 1994.

34. Josephson ME: Surgical and nonsurgical ablation in the therapy of arrhythmias, in Josephson ME (ed): *Clinical Cardiac Electrophysiology Techniques and Interpretations,* ed 2. Philadelphia, Lea & Febiger, 1993, p 803.

CHAPTER 7

Perioperative Cardiac Imaging

Solomon Aronson, MD, FCCP
Associate Professor, Department of Anesthesia and Critical Care,
University of Chicago; Director of Cardiothoracic Anesthesia, University
of Chicago Hospitals, Chicago, Illinois

Frank W. Dupont, MD
Clinical Associate, Department of Anesthesia and Critical Care,
University of Chicago, University of Chicago Hospitals, Chicago, Illinois

Since its clinical introduction and initial slow growth during the 1950s and 1960s, cardiac ultrasound application and utilization has rapidly expanded. During the last decade in particular, progress in the techniques of diagnostic ultrasound imaging has been fast and furious. The application and validation of these ultrasound technologies to the perioperative arena have and should continue to greatly affect patient care and the role of the perioperative specialist. In this chapter we will review some of the most recent and important advances in ultrasound technology in global and regional ventricular function monitoring and the distinct but interrelated ultrasound area of myocardial perfusion assessment.

ASSESSMENT OF GLOBAL VENTRICULAR FUNCTION

Assessment of global and regional ventricular function has become the cornerstone for evaluating patients with ischemic heart disease. The dynamic assessment of global ventricular function is based on echocardiographic-derived indices of muscle contraction, relaxation, and filling, which are obtained from analysis of moving images. Echocardiography is therefore inherently a qualitative technique and as such, does not ordinarily provide quantitative values for common indices of global left ventricular (LV) systolic function.

When using transesophageal echocardiography (TEE) to evaluate global ventricular systolic function, one is really attempting to make inferences about a 3-dimensional structure from 2-dimensional measurements. To do so, either images must be acquired in multiple planes, or assumptions (explicitly or implicitly) must be made about the shape of the ventricle. Echocardiographic parameters can be derived from endocardial border outlines and a combination of Doppler techniques to assess preload, contractility, afterload, and parameters of ventricular relaxation and filling.

ASSESSMENT OF PRELOAD

Preload can be assessed through the evaluation of LV end-diastolic area (EDA) or LV end-diastolic pressure. Both can be estimated from TEE. When echocardiography is used for evaluation of LV areas, the transgastric short-axis view at the midpapillary should be used. Good correlation has been found between the transgastric short-axis view obtained with TEE and radionuclide imaging in the estimation of LV volume. Despite variable loading conditions, changes in LV short-axis area have been shown to reflect changes in LV volume.[1,2] The ability to see the intraventricular cavity allows a rapid way to appreciate volume status, independent of LV pressure or compliance factors. A decrease in EDA (<5.5 cm^2/m^2) invariably reflects hypovolemia. However, setting an upper limit of EDA below which hypovolemia can be confirmed is difficult. This is particularly true in patients with impaired contractility or acute afterload elevations where a compensatory baseline increase in preload makes the echocardiographic diagnosis of hypovolemia difficult.

Pulmonary venous flow as measured by pulsed-wave Doppler echocardiography can be used to assess left atrial pressure (LAP). In using this technique, the flow recording is compared with a simultaneous electrocardiography (ECG) tracing so that the systolic and diastolic peaks can be identified and their respective velocity-time integral measurements can be performed. When LAP is less than 15 mm Hg, the pulmonary venous flow velocities are predominant in systole. Increases in LAP (>15 mm Hg) have been shown to result in a shift of higher flow velocities toward early diastole.[3]

ASSESSMENT OF SYSTOLIC FUNCTION

The ability to judge volumes by 2-dimensional area analysis allows the determination of LV systolic function indices such as the ejection fraction. Determination of the fractional area change (FAC) can be calculated from end-systolic area (ESA) and EDA, obtained from the transgastric short-axis view at the midpapillary level, with the following formula:

$$FAC\% = EDA–ESA/EDA \times 100$$

whereby EDA is synchronized to the R wave on the ECG, and ESA is synchronized to the dicrotic notch on the arterial pressure tracing or the time of smallest LV diameter at the middle of the T wave. Its value in individuals with normal LV function varies from 50% to 75%. Good correlation has been found between 2-dimensional TEE derived FAC and ejection fraction determined from other techniques.[4] Echocardiographic automated border detection appears to be a promising new means of rapid on-line determination of LV dimensions that give reliable information about areas and FAC when compared with manual tracing.[5]

With automated border detection, volume versus time relationships during systole and diastole can be compared. In addition, LV end-systolic pressure–volume relations have been proposed as load-independent indices of contractile function. The combination of continuous volume-dimension assessment with automatic border detection together with pressure data acquisition has enabled the generation of end-systolic pressure-volume loops.[5]

In addition, the assessment of right and left heart function can be accomplished with intraoperative echocardiography. The assessment of right heart damage and left heart damage during intraoperative ischemia monitoring is essential because the presence of right ventricular (RV) dysfunction may be a limiting factor and thus influence perioperative treatment strategies.[6,7]

ASSESSMENT OF AFTERLOAD

TEE when used together with ventricular pressure measurements can provide an accurate measure of wall stress, by enabling an estimation of wall thickness and LV diameter. End-systolic wall stress (ESWS) can be calculated as follows:

$$ESWS = \frac{1.33 \times pd}{4th\ (1+h/d)}$$

where p is the peak intra-arterial pressure (or LV end-systolic pressure), d is the internal diameter of the ventricle, and h is the wall thickness.

Reichert et al[8] showed that the systolic arterial pressure obtained noninvasively with a blood pressure cuff can be substituted for the

LV end-systolic pressure if a correcting factor is used (LV end-systolic pressure = 0.89 × systolic arterial pressure, ± 8.1) in the absence of significant mitral regurgitation. In healthy individuals, the ESWS is equal to approximately 65×10^3 dynes/cm^2.

ASSESSMENT OF DIASTOLIC FUNCTION

Alteration in LV diastolic function may result from systolic dysfunction or, in as many as 40% of patients, may present as the primary and main etiology of cardiac failure. Abnormalities of diastolic function may precede those of systolic dysfunction and be an early marker of disease.

Evaluation of diastolic function implies that we are able to assess the pressure-volume relationship of LV diastolic filling. This relationship can only be measured hemodynamically. Doppler echocardiography attempts to evaluate diastolic filling by evaluating patterns and timing of flow, such as from the left atrium into the left ventricle or the pulmonary veins into the left atrium. The main determination of flow is the pressure difference between the two chambers; however, other factors such as chamber size, compliance, LV loading conditions, RV and LV interaction, and a pericardial constraint can also influence rates of LV filling.

LV diastolic function can be assessed by pulsed Doppler interrogation of mitral valve and pulmonary venous inflow velocities in the midesophageal 4-chamber view (Fig 1).[9] The transmitral velocity has 2 peaks: an early filling (E) peak and a later lower (A) peak associated with atrial contraction. The pulmonary venous inflow pattern reveals systolic (S wave), diastolic (D wave), and atrial (A wave) components. When impaired relaxation is present, early diastolic transmitral filling is reduced (decreased E), atrial filling is increased (increased A), and the ratio (E/A) decreases. Pulmonary venous diastolic filling of the left atrium may also be reduced because of the delayed atrial emptying. As diastolic function worsens, left atrial pressure may rise, increasing early transmitral diastolic pressure and leading to an increased E velocity and normalization of the mitral inflow patterns. Pseudonormalized filling can be confusing because the mitral inflow pattern can appear normal. A clue may be upper-normal E velocities and relatively short deceleration time. Unmasking pseudonormalization requires evaluation of pulmonary venous flow, performance of the Valsalva maneuver, or both. In this situation, LV end-diastolic pressure is usually elevated. When this is the case, left atrial blood will reflux into the pulmonary veins at end-diastole, resulting in an increase in pulmonary venous A wave

Diastolic Filling Mitral Inflow Common Patterns

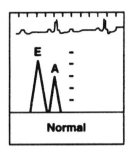
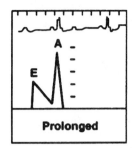
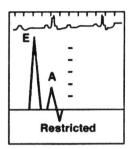

Diastolic Filling Pulmonary Vein Common Patterns

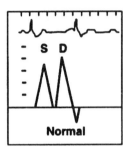
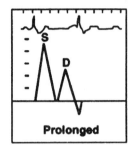
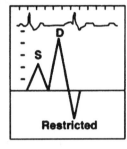

FIGURE 1.
Pulsed Doppler mitral inflow and pulmonary venous inflow patterns. *Abbreviations: E,* Early filling peak; *A,* peak associated with atrial contraction; *S,* systolic; *D,* diastolic.

reversal. By reducing the pressure difference between the left atrium and left ventricle, the Valsalva maneuver unmasks E/A reversal.

REGIONAL VENTRICULAR FUNCTION AND ISCHEMIA DETECTION

The relationship of echocardiographic indices of regional myocardial function to ischemia has been compared with changes that occur with surface ECG, pulmonary capillary wedge pressure (PCWP), and the onset of chest pain. As early as 1935, it was recognized that acute myocardial ischemia results in abnormal inward motion and thickening of the affected myocardial region.[10] Since then, wall motion abnormalities have been shown to occur within seconds of inadequate blood flow or oxygen supply.[11] These abnormal contraction patterns typically occur at the same time as regional lactate production.[12,13]

The precise sequence of regional functional changes that occurs in the myocardium after interruption of flow has been studied in models of acute ischemia, including percutaneous transluminal coronary angioplasty.[14-16] Systolic function is estimated qualitatively and is reflected echocardiographically by regional wall thickening and wall motion during systole. Systolic wall thickening can be calculated from the equation:

$$PSWT = SWT - DWT/SWT \times 100$$

where *PSWT* is the percentage systolic wall thickening, *SWT* is the end-systolic wall thickness, and *DWT* is the end-diastolic wall thickness (Fig 2). Regional wall motion is characterized by observing the movement of the endocardium during systole. As the myocardial oxygen supply to demand balance worsens, graded regional wall motion abnormalities progress from mild hypokinesia to severe hypokinesia, akinesia, and finally dyskinesia.[10,17] Hypokinesia refers to inward contraction that is slower and less vigorous than normal during systole. Severe hypokinesia is an extreme example of hypokinesia, whereas mild hypokinesia may appear to be quite subtle compared with normal inward contraction. The precise distinction between varying degrees of hypokinesia can be difficult. Akinesia refers to the absence of wall motion or no inward movement of the endocardium during systole. Dyskinesia refers to paradoxical wall motion or movement outward during ventricular systole (Table 1).

Clinical studies have indicated that abnormal changes in segmental wall motion occur earlier and are a more sensitive indica-

End-diastole   End-systole

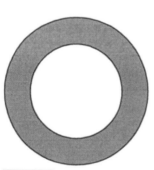 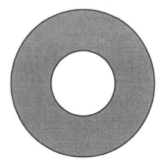

FIGURE 2.
Systolic wall thickening.

TABLE 1.

Classes of Segmental Wall Motion Abnormalities

Class of Motion	Wall Thickening	Change in Radius
Normal	Marked	>30% ↓
Mild hypokinesis	Moderate	10%-30% ↓
Severe hypokinesis	Minimal	<10%, >0% ↓
Akinesis	None	None
Dyskinesis	Thinning	↑

tor of myocardial ischemia than the abnormal changes detected with an ECG[12,18-21] or pulmonary artery catheter.[22-24] In one study,[21] 30 patients undergoing percutaneous transluminal coronary angioplasty were simultaneously monitored with 12-lead ECGs and echocardiography. All the patients had isolated obstructive lesions in their left anterior descending coronary arteries, stable angina, normal baseline ECGs, and normal baseline myocardial function with no prior history of infarction and no angiographic evidence of collateralization. In the study, all patients had segmental wall motion abnormalities (SWMAs) approximately 10 seconds after coronary artery occlusion, and 27 of the 30 had repolarization changes in their ECGs at approximately 22 seconds.

Smith et al[20] evaluated 50 patients at high risk for myocardial ischemia during peripheral vascular or cardiac surgery with TEE, multilead ECG, and a 12-lead ECG. In their study, 6 patients had repolarization changes diagnostic of ischemia, whereas 24 had new evidence of SWMAs. SWMAs occurred minutes before ECG changes in 3 of these 6 patients, and no ST-segment change occurred before or without new SWMAs. Three patients who sustained intraoperative myocardial infarctions (MIs) had SWMAs in the corresponding area of myocardium that persisted until the end of surgery, but only 1 of these 3 had ischemic ST-segment changes intraoperatively. Four of 5 patients with double-vessel disease had SWMAs in regions of myocardium supplied by the diseased coronary arteries, never in the "risk-free" myocardium. Neither SWMAs nor ST-segment changes occurred in the 10 other study patients without coronary disease. Subsequent studies in comparable patients (ie, those undergoing coronary artery bypass surgery) confirmed these initial findings.

The value of PCWP monitoring for ischemia has also been compared with changes in regional LV function assessed with TEE. In one study, PCWP, 12-lead ECG, and LV wall motion were evaluated in 98 patients before coronary artery bypass grafting (CABG), at predetermined intervals.[22] Myocardial ischemia was diagnosed by TEE in 14 patients. In 10 of the 14 patients, ischemia was associated with repolarization changes on the ECG. An increase of at least 3 mm Hg in PCWP was tested as an indicator for ischemia and was sensitive only 33% of the time, with a positive predictive value of only 16%. Overall, most studies indicate that the sensitivity of wall motion analysis for the detection of myocardial ischemia is generally superior to that of ECG or PCWP monitoring.

Although TEE appears to have many advantages over traditional intraoperative monitors of myocardial ischemia, there remain potential limitations as well. The most obvious limitation of TEE monitoring is that ischemia cannot be detected during critical periods such as induction, laryngoscopy, intubation, emergence, and extubation. In addition, the adequacy of wall motion analysis may be influenced by artifacts (Table 2).[25] Artifacts can be produced by the ultrasound system itself or by the particular tangential section being imaged. The septum in particular must be given special consideration with respect to wall motion and wall thickness assessment.[25-27] The septum is composed of two parts, the lower muscular portion and the basal membranous portion. The basal septum does not exhibit the same degree of contraction as the lower muscular part. At the most superior basal portion the septum is attached to the aortic outflow track. Its movement at this level is normally paradoxical during ventricular systole. The septum is also a unique region of the left ventricle, because it is a region of the right ventricle as well, and is therefore influenced by forces from both ventricles. In addition, sternotomy, pericardiotomy, and cardiopulmonary bypass (CPB) have been suggested to alter the translational and rotational motion of the heart within the chest that may cause changes in ventricular septal motion.[27]

TABLE 2.
Artifacts Affecting SWMA Analysis

Cross-section
Dropout
Conduction abnormality
V-pacing
Cardiac tamponade

Abbreviation: SWMA, Segmental wall motion abnormality.

Consequently, the exact imaging plane for wall motion assessment is critical. The short-axis view of the left ventricle at the level of the midpapillary muscles is used to ensure constant internal landmarks as reference (anterolateral and posteromedial papillary muscles) and to ensure monitoring of the muscular septal region. It must be recognized that although myocardial blood flow from the coronary arteries is best represented at the short-axis midpapillary muscle level, there may be other myocardial regions that are underperfused and not adequately represented in one echocardiographic imaging plane.[28] One solution to this problem is to frequently reposition the probe to view other cross-sections of the heart. Another potential problem of wall motion assessment is evaluation of the discoordinated contraction that occurs because of bundle-branch block or ventricular pacing. In this situation, the system used to assess SWMAs must compensate for global motion of the heart (usually done with a floating frame of reference) and evaluate not only regional endocardial wall motion but myocardial thickening as well.

Not all SWMAs are indicative of myocardial ischemia or infarction (Table 3). Clearly, under normal conditions, all hearts do not contract in a homogeneous and consistent manner.[29] It is reasonable to assume, however, that most of the time an acute change in the regional contraction pattern of the heart during surgery is likely attributable to myocardial ischemia. An important exception to this rule may apply in models of acute coronary artery occlusion. In these models, myocardial function becomes abnormal not only in the center of an ischemic zone, but also in myocardial regions adjacent to the ischemic zone. Several studies have reported that the total area of dysfunctional myocardium commonly exceeds the area of ischemic or infarcted myocardium.[30,31] The impairment of

TABLE 3.
Differential Diagnosis of SWMAs

Ischemia
Infarction
Hibernation
Stunning
Conduction abnormality
Loading condition
Tethering

Abbreviation: SWMA, Segmental wall motion abnormalities.

TABLE 4.
Nonischemic Causes of SWMAs

Stunning
Tethering
Unmasking loading changes
Artifacts

Abbreviation: SWMAs, Segmental wall motion abnormalities.

function in nonischemic tissue has been thought to be caused by a tethering effect. Tethering, or the attachment of noncontracting tissue that mechanically impairs contraction in normally perfused adjacent tissue, probably accounts for the consistent overestimation of infarct size by echocardiography when compared with findings from postmortem studies.[32] Another limitation of SWMA analysis during surgery is that it does not differentiate stunned or hibernating myocardium from acute ischemia,[33] nor does it differentiate the cause of ischemia between increased oxygen demand or decreased oxygen supply. Finally, it should be noted that areas of previous ischemia or scarring may become unmasked by changes in afterload and appear as new SWMAs (Table 4).[34]

Data regarding the significance of intraoperative detection of SWMAs suggest that transient abnormalities unaccompanied by hemodynamic or ECG evidence of ischemia may not represent clinically significant myocardial ischemia and are usually not associated with postoperative morbidity.[35] The significance of the severity of SWMAs has been studied.[11,15] Hypokinetic myocardial segments appear to be associated with minimal perfusion defects compared with significant perfusion defects that accompany akinetic or dyskinetic segments. Hence, hypokinesia may be a less-predictive marker for postoperative morbidity than akinesis or dyskinesis. Persistent severe SWMAs on the other hand are clearly associated with myocardial ischemia and postoperative morbidity.[20,36-38]

Intraoperative detection of new or worsened and persistent SWMAs during peripheral vascular surgery has been reported to be associated with postoperative cardiac morbidity by several investigators. The occurrence of new segmental wall motion changes during vascular surgery appear to be common[35-38]; however, most of the time they are transient and clinically insignificant. New SWMAs that are recognized to persist until the conclusion of surgery, on the other hand, imply perioperative acute

MI.[20,35-38] Intraoperative wall motion abnormalities, therefore, may be spurious, reversible with or without treatment, or irreversible. The former may be associated with clinically insignificant short periods of ischemia, whereas the latter is associated with significant ischemia or infarction.

Two-dimensional TEE has been shown to greatly enhance the diagnostic potential for detecting life-threatening sequelae of MI such as ruptured ventricular septum or ruptured papillary muscles.[39,40] It has also been recognized that TEE may enable the identification of subtle but potentially significant problems that complicate the management of ischemic heart disease, such as anomalous coronary artery origins[41] and atrial infarction. The detection of iatrogenically introduced intracardiac air after cardiac surgery is greatly enhanced with intraoperative TEE,[42,43] and may be used to guide "de-airing" strategies.

During CABG, TEE has helped predict the results of surgery. After CABG to previously dysfunctional segments, immediate improvement of regional myocardial function (which is sustained) has been demonstrated.[44,45] In addition, prebypass compensatory hypercontracting segments have been reported to revert toward normal immediately after successful CABG.[46] Persistent SWMAs after CABG appear to be related to adverse clinical outcomes, whereas lack of evidence of SWMAs after CABG has been shown to be associated with a postoperative course without cardiac morbidity.[23]

ASSESSMENT OF MYOCARDIAL VIABILITY

The perioperative diagnosis of viability (Table 5) after an acute ischemic insult (stunned myocardium)[33] has traditionally been based on clinical signs of an "incomplete" MI such as a small cre-

---

TABLE 5.

Diagnostic Techniques for the Assessment of Myocardial Viability

---

ECG: Q waves
ECHO: SWMAs
Nuclear: myocardial cell membrane function
DSE: contractile reserve
MCE: microvascular integrity
PET: myocardial metabolism

Abbreviations: ECG, Electrocardiography; *ECHO,* echocardiography; *SWMA,* segmental wall motion abnormalities; *DSE,* dobutamine stress echocardiography; *MCE,* myocardial contrast echocardiography; *PET,* positron emission tomography.

atine phosphokinase leak or non–Q wave ECG changes. In patients with chronic coronary artery disease who harbor hibernating myocardium,[47] evidence of preserved wall thickness (with resting echocardiography) within a hypocontractile region has been a clue to viability. Positron emission tomography (PET) scanning, the gold standard for such assessment, uses regional markers of glucose metabolism to demonstrate viability and functional recovery, whereas radionuclear imaging techniques are predicated on cellular membrane function for perfusion data. Current radionuclear imaging techniques with newer agents may also provide functional information and can be combined with inotropic and vasodilator agents. Studies have shown up to a 40% rate of discordance between PET evidence of viability and these other modalities for determining the need for coronary revascularization.[48] Neither PET scanning nor radionuclide imaging techniques, however, are practical for intraoperative assessment of viability.

Reversible postoperative ventricular contractile dysfunction that is unrelated to a continuing source of ischemia (ie, myocardial stunning) has been reported to occur after CABG surgery.[49] Distinguishing ventricular dysfunction caused by inadequate flow (ongoing ischemia or infarction) from reversible contractile dysfunction (stunned myocardium) remains critical for determining long-term prognosis and perioperative management strategies (Fig 3).[33,50-52] Improvement in regional function after an acute MI or ischemic event has been reported to occur up to 3 weeks after the initial compromising episode, despite adequate restoration of coronary blood flow.[33,49] Contractile reserve (the augmented contractile function of a dyssynergic segment) has been demonstrated with dobutamine stress echocardiography (DSE).[53] Myocardial contrast echocardiography (MCE), on the other hand, provides evidence of intact microcirculation and perfusion. Both techniques can be easily used in the operating room suite and when combined, provide evidence of different myocardial viability states. Understanding how to identify reversible contractile dysfunction conditions (eg, stunning, hibernation, and silent ischemia) is critical during ischemic heart surgery for optimal revascularization. The combined use of MCE and DSE in the operating room should provide evidence of perfusion-contraction mismatching and contractile reserve. The ability of these techniques in combination during surgery to provide data for predicting improved functional recovery after revascularization or therapeutic intervention has not yet been studied.

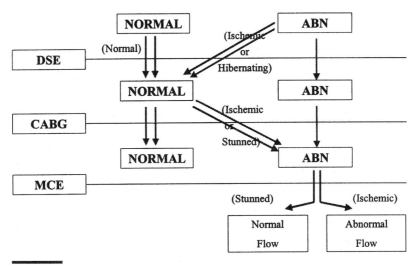

FIGURE 3.

Intraoperative assessment of myocardial function during coronary artery bypass graft *(CABG)* surgery. *Abbreviations: DSE,* Dobutamine stress echocardiography; *ABN,* abnormal; *MCE,* myocardial contrast echocardiography.

DSE

Preoperative LV systolic function is among the most powerful predictors of perioperative morbidity and mortality,[54] and regional wall motion abnormalities contribute prominently to LV dysfunction.[50,55] In patients with coronary artery disease, dysfunctional myocardium at rest may represent either infarcted or viable myocardium.[33,47,56] Resting 2-dimensional echocardiography, a commonly used imaging modality to detect regional ventricular dysfunction, cannot differentiate acute dysfunction but viable myocardium (eg, stunned myocardium) or chronic and reversible dysfunction (hibernating myocardium) from irreversibly damaged myocardium, because it does not account for coronary blood flow reserve. Because regional LV dysfunction is often reversible and exists in territories of viable myocardium,[44,50,57] provocative testing is necessary to diagnose ischemic and viable segments. During the past decade, stress echocardiography has emerged as a safe and sensitive method for the detection of coronary artery disease and a cost-efficient alternative to other imaging modalities, such as scintigraphy, and it has been used to provide data for risk stratification during the perioperative period.[58-60]

Common pharmacologic regimens used during stress echocardiography are dobutamine, dobutamine with atropine, dipyridamole, and adenosine. These techniques have been demonstrated to be safe, with sensitivity and specificity rivaling thallium-201 exercise scintigraphy.[61] Of these agents, dobutamine is the most extensively studied. Dobutamine is a racemic mixture of enantiomers with α_1, β_1, and β_2 effects and a half-life of about 2 minutes.[62] The α_1 and β_1 effects are responsible for inotropism independent of endogenous norepinephrine stores.[62] The response of regional LV function to dobutamine is useful to characterize myocardial reserve capacity (Fig 4). In the therapeutic dose range (5-20 μg/kg per min), cardiac output is augmented by an increase in ventricular contractility, heart rate, and stroke volume, and a β_2-mediated decrease in systemic vascular resistance. Contractility increases at higher doses (20-40 μg/kg per min).

Normal resting wall motion and the development of hyperdynamic function with increasing doses of dobutamine are hallmarks of normally perfused myocardium.[63-65] The development of new

CORONARY BLOOD FLOW

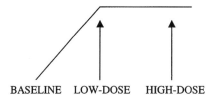

BASELINE   LOW-DOSE   HIGH-DOSE

REGIONAL OXYGEN DEMAND

BASELINE   LOW-DOSE   HIGH-DOSE

FIGURE 4.
Low- and high-dose dobutamine effect on coronary blood flow and regional oxygen demand.

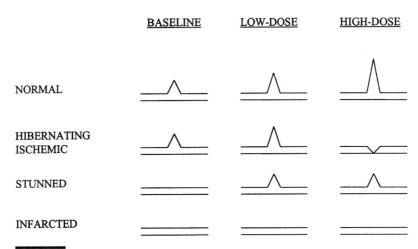

FIGURE 5.
Pre-CABG dobutamine dose response. *Abbreviation: CABG,* Coronary artery bypass graft.

wall motion abnormalities or the worsening of baseline systolic dysfunction with escalating doses of dobutamine indicates myocardial ischemia. Contractile reserve, on the other hand, is consistent with viability and characterized by baseline wall motion abnormalities that improve with low-dose dobutamine.[63,64,66] When such a low-dose augmentation of function is followed by progressive systolic dysfunction with higher doses (biphasic response), the accuracy of predicting postoperative cardiac morbidity or changes in regional function after revascularization is enhanced.[66] Regional segments that remain akinetic or dyskinetic despite dobutamine infusion are nonviable and likely reflect scar (Fig 5). We often only infuse low-dose dobutamine to augment baseline coronary blood flow and assess the changes in regional myocardial function reserve to be used as a gold standard to predict the myocardial flow-function relationship after revascularization.

The patients' regional function should be evaluated with intraoperative TEE imaging in the transgastric midpapillary short-axis, midesophageal 4-chamber, 2-chamber, and long-axis view using a multiplane transducer. Semiquantitative analysis of echocardiographic images is based on a standard 16-segment model of the left ventricle (Fig 6). Each segment is scored on a 4-point scale according to the methods of the American Society of Echocardiography.[67] In the LV short-axis view, the left coronary artery territory will extend from the anterior septum to the posterolateral wall. The anterior septum and anterior wall will typically be the left anterior descending territory, whereas the lateral and posterior walls will be the circumflex artery territory. The right coronary territory will include the inferior wall and septum (Fig 6).

There are several studies comparing dobutamine, adenosine, and dipyridamole as stressors. In a crossover, blind, comparative

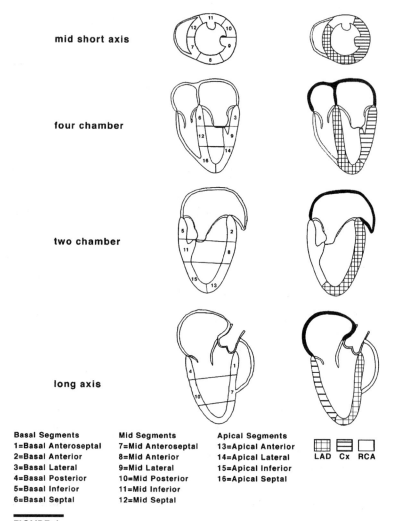

mid short axis

four chamber

two chamber

long axis

Basal Segments	Mid Segments	Apical Segments
1=Basal Anteroseptal	7=Mid Anteroseptal	13=Apical Anterior
2=Basal Anterior	8=Mid Anterior	14=Apical Lateral
3=Basal Lateral	9=Mid Lateral	15=Apical Inferior
4=Basal Posterior	10=Mid Posterior	16=Apical Septal
5=Basal Inferior	11=Mid Inferior	
6=Basal Septal	12=Mid Septal	

LAD   Cx   RCA

FIGURE 6.
Sixteen-segment model of the left ventricle for segmental wall motion abnormalities—analysis and coronary blood supply. *Abbreviations: LAD,* Left anterior descending; *Cx,* circumflex; *RCA,* right coronary artery.

study,[68] dobutamine was tolerated best of the three agents with the unique advantage of incremental infusion during the protocol. Increasing the dose gradually to a maximum rate of 0.04 mg/kg approximates physiologic responses to exercise and allows evaluation of ischemic changes in a dose-related fashion. DSE has a high sensitivity (85%) and specificity (88%) when compared with angiography in patients with recent MI.[69] A meta-analysis of data from several studies revealed overall sensitivity and specificity of the test for detecting ischemic heart disease to be 82% and 86%, respectively.[62] A recent review of echocardiographic data for the assessment of myocardial viability[56] reported that dobutamine echocardiography is slightly more specific than thallium scintigraphy at predicting recovery of regional function after an ischemic event; however, sensitivity is slightly less. A possible explanation is that a higher level of myocyte functional integrity is necessary for demonstration of contractile reserve by dobutamine echocardiography than for evidence of intact membrane function necessary for thallium uptake. Furthermore, it has been demonstrated that changes in wall motion in the setting of an increased heart rate and low filling pressure[70] may not reflect myocardial ischemia and further reduce the specificity of DSE prediction of risk and functional recovery.

Stress echocardiography has been shown to be an efficient method for identifying patients undergoing major vascular surgery who are at high or low risk of perioperative cardiac events.[71] DSE has been used to distinguish hibernating myocardium from nonviable myocardium before revascularization by identifying patients with severe LV dysfunction who had improved regional wall thickening with dobutamine infusion.[72] More than 80% of these patients had improved regional LV wall thickening after revascularization.

The application of stress echocardiography intraoperatively may allow for on-line identification of the extent of myocardial salvage and viability during coronary revascularization surgery. The ability to differentiate intraoperatively the clinical scenarios of ischemia or infarction of the myocardium from stunning or hibernation of the myocardium can help to define inadequate myocardial revascularization and the need for revision of the surgical plan or other therapeutic options during coronary bypass surgery, thereby allowing more efficient utilization of resources (eg, return to bypass, utilization of a mechanical assist device, administration of vasoactive drugs) to improve the quality of care and decrease costs. For example, because the postischemic myocardium has contractile reserve, an inotrope such as dobuta-mine should increase wall thickening in viable but otherwise stunned myocardium. When myocardial necrosis coexists with stunned myocardium, dobutamine echocardiography can be used to determine the amount of tissue that has escaped necrosis.

No studies have addressed whether the identification and revas-cularization of dysfunctional but viable myocardium improves patient outcomes. Barilla et al,[73] however, reported that patients with viable myocardium treated medically had less recovery of LV systolic function than those who were revascularized. Voci et al[74] showed that microvascular revascularization improves functional outcome. Also of note has been the poor outcome (48% average event rate during 12- to 36-month follow-up periods) noted in patients with viable myocardium when these regions were not revascularized.[75,76] The high rate of cardiac events was signifi-cantly lower (11%-16%) in patients with viable segments that were revascularized. Unfortunately, many techniques to assess revascularization only provide anatomical evidence of vessel patency rather than microvascular flow into the tissue at risk. Therefore, studies that compare long-term functional recovery out-come and revascularization are limited in their capacity to assess true microvascular integrity.

Currently, preoperative screening tests are expensive and time-consuming, often causing delay of surgery and contributing to patient dissatisfaction. Nevertheless, understanding information regarding the extent of the patient's cardiovascular disease is use-ful in tailoring optimal perioperative strategies for care. Many investigators have demonstrated the utility of preoperative provocative myocardial testing for long-term risk stratification. Based on these data, decisions are often made regarding intraoper-ative management choices and postoperative disposition. Data support that prolonged and intensive monitoring after high-risk surgery in high-risk patients is associated with reduced cardiovas-cular morbidity. The use of such intensive medical therapy and monitoring, however, is associated with risks, costs, and utiliza-tion of scarce resources. Because there is increasing pressure to minimize cost and delays for preoperative patient evaluation, intraoperative stress echocardiography may be particularly well suited for use in patients who have known coronary artery disease or who are at high risk of postoperative cardiac morbidity. An intraoperative paradigm that demonstrates postoperative outcome benefits and thereby enables more efficient utilization and alloca-tion of otherwise scarce resources (eg, ICU beds) is likely to improve quality of care and reduce cost. However, although monitoring high-risk patients with intraoperative echocardiography is routine at most institutions, the dose-response relationship between preoperative DSE, physiology of coronary flow reserve coupled to myocardial oxygen demand, and long-term outcome is not known. Before extrapolation of risk stratification data of intraoperative DSE testing can be unequivocally applied to perioperative decision analysis, the dose-response relationship of intraoperative DSE to preoperative DSE should be understood.

MCE

The clinical need to directly assess the quality and quantity of blood supply to the heart intraoperatively is not satisfied by traditional monitoring techniques. During cardiac surgery for ischemic heart disease, assessment of myocardial perfusion remains the goal to provide information for assurance of unobstructed graft and anastomotic sites, appropriate selection of target vessels, adequate myocardial reperfusion, and improved functional recovery after revascularization. Toward that goal, several techniques have been used. Probing anastomosis, measuring graft blood flow with electromagnetic flowmeters, and using high-frequency echo transducers to assess flow velocity through grafts have been used to provide information about the integrity of the anastomosis site.[77] Probing anastomosis or stripping grafts may cause damage to vessel endothelium, and moreover, measurement of graft blood flow by these methods as well as flowmeter or Doppler echocardiography techniques does not provide evidence about regional myocardial perfusion in the revascularized myocardium. Among the methods available to measure regional myocardial perfusion, such as PET scanning, ultrafast CT, radionuclear imaging, and contrast echocardiography,[78] it appears that only MCE is practical for application in the operating room setting.

MCE is a diagnostic technique that uses an ultrasound contrast agent and adapted ultrasound systems to enhance ultrasound imaging and provide a safe, noninvasive means of directly assessing myocardial perfusion. Compared with other imaging modalities, MCE is relatively inexpensive (provided an ultrasound machine is present), user friendly, and portable, making it an excellent option for the operative setting. Important information such as the adequacy of myocardial revascularization after CABG surgery, the efficacy of myocardial protection as a consequence of homogenous distribution of cardioplegia solution, the extent of collateral myocardial circulation subserved by native and saphenous vein bypass vessels, and the effect of therapy on transmural distribution of myocardial blood flow has been demonstrated with contrast ultrasonography techniques during cardiac surgery, and will be reviewed.

Assessment of Myocardial Revascularization

MCE is a technique used to assess the integrity of the coronary microcirculation. The visualization of microbubbles by this technique assesses flow through vessels with diameters of less than 100 µg and provides evidence for microvascular integrity, which is a marker for viability. The first experience with contrast ultrasonography for evaluating myocardial revascularization during surgery was reported by Kabas et al[79] in 1990.

Assessment of myocardial perfusion with contrast ultrasonography from aortic root injections was later reported.[80,81] Aronson et al[81] reported delineation of changes in regional myocardial blood flow before, during, and after CABG surgery using TEE to obtain tomographic myocardial images. In that study, Renografin-76 was injected into the cardioplegia line routinely placed into the aortic root (prebypass grafting) to identify myocardial regions with compromised flow. In addition, selective injections of contrast were made into the proximal end of each saphenous vein graft after completion of the distal anastomosis. Injections directly into saphenous veins provided information about the magnitude and geometric distribution of new-vessel flow into the heart. After the completion of all coronary artery–vein bypass grafts, contrast was again injected into the aortic root during warm-blood reperfusion through the cardioplegia line. These postbypass injections allowed the identification of myocardial regions that remained poorly perfused before separation from CPB. It was subsequently recognized that areas with perfusion deficits before separation from CPB were correlated to regions with wall motion abnormalities after separation from CPB. When predicted myocardial perfusion patterns (based on preoperative angiograms) were compared with actual perfusion patterns assessed from intraoperative contrast studies, predicted patterns were actualized 84% of the time.

Application of intraoperative MCE for assessment of appropriateness of target site and reperfusion after revascularization should ideally provide information at the time of the operation. Villanueva et al[82] compared an on-line analysis of echocardiographic information with off-line visual assessment during coronary bypass graft operations. Twenty-one patients with multivessel disease were studied with epicardial and transesophageal imaging. Analogue images were digitized, and video-intensity in each region of interest was measured in real time. Contrast enhancement was assessed before and after bypass in 17 of the 21 patients. Quantitative assessment agreed with visual assessment in 91% of their comparisons. Furthermore, analysis of myocardial perfusion before and after grafting showed three distinct patterns of contrast enhancement. The first pattern showed reduced contrast before and improved after grafting; the second pattern showed adequate contrast before and no change after; and the third pattern showed no contrast before or after. The latter was associated with an old inferior MI.

In another study by Mudra et al,[83] 12 patients undergoing coronary bypass surgery were evaluated with quantitative MCE and epicardial imaging. Videodensitometry was used, and images were analyzed for contrast delay half time and peak pixel intensity after injection of sonicated lobromid into the left main coronary artery, the saphenous vein grafts, or both. They reported that MCE visualized native and bypass-dependent myocardial perfusion immediately after insertion of the graft and identified adequacy of revascularization. The availability of commercially produced ultrasound contrast agents has greatly enhanced the ease of application of this technique.[84]

In another application, Jacobsohn et al[85] used Albunex to demonstrate regional myocardial perfusion after an internal mammary artery to left anterior descending artery anastomosis during minimally invasive coronary bypass surgery. This application provided on-line evidence of graft patency and adequacy of revascularization in this technically challenging procedure, thereby obviating the need for confirmation with angiography. In general, assessment of the perfusion bed supplied by the internal mammary artery has been fleeting. Spotnitz et al[86] reported a technique in the canine model for demonstrating the adequacy of internal mammary artery bypassing; however, their results have not been realized in clinical practice. We have also demonstrated in the laboratory the potential to perfuse the left internal mammary artery distribution bed during coronary bypass surgery and CPB with retrograde injection of contrast immediately before release of the occlusive clamp after coronary anastomosis. Our results, however, have also been difficult to reproduce clinically. It appears that the newer contrast agents which obviate the need for direct, intra-arterial injection will overcome these limitations in this unique and important vascular bed.

The assessment of transmural distribution of flow by means of MCE during coronary bypass surgery has been reported. Hirata et al[87] reported regional perfusion and transmural blood flow distribution changes after revascularization in 31 patients. Injection of 5% human albumin into saphenous vein grafts was performed along with off-line videodensitometry to demonstrate endocardial to epicardial distribution of flow in revascularized regions.

Finally, the relationship between function and flow has been evaluated in patients with coronary artery disease by contrast echocardiography. In patients with acute MI and occlusion of the infarct-related artery, the presence of collateral flow by MCE correlated with improvement in regional wall motion 1 month after successful coronary angioplasty.[88] A subsequent study showed that in patients with documented patency of the infarct-related artery after recent MI, there was a strong correlation between evidence of an intact microcirculation and subsequent improvement in regional wall motion. During acute MI, patients with evidence of reflow by MCE in the myocardial area at risk after reperfusion therapy had greater improvement in global and regional LV function on follow-up than patients with no reflow.[89] With respect to chronic ischemia, perfusion by MCE correlated with improvement in regional wall motion and global LV function after revascularization in a population of patients with previous MI and reduced LV ejection fraction.[90] Aronson et al[91] used intraoperative MCE to identify the cause of LV systolic dysfunction after coronary bypass surgery and determine the relationship between flow and function after CABG surgery. In that study, MCE opacification of flow was graded from intraoperative TEE images of the left ventricle in the short-axis midpapillary view (Fig 7). The same myocardial images were also evaluated for regional wall motion abnormalities at 15, 30, and 60 minutes, 24 hours, 7 days, and 1 month after CPB. Logistic regression analysis was used to analyze the flow scores and regional function data from identical segments. Regional flow represented by contrast enhancement was assessed in 70% of the myocardial regions. Regional myocardial contrast flow patterns did not predict regional myocardial function at 15, 30, or 60 minutes after separation from CPB. However, contrast opacification of flow did predict regional myocardial function at 1 week ($P \le .05$) and at 1 month ($P \le .01$) after CABG surgery. The probability that myocardial function would be normal at 1 month was 0.62 when intraoperative flow opacification was abnormal and 0.98 when flow opacification was normal. For patients with normal flow, the estimated odds of having normal myocardial function were 3.33

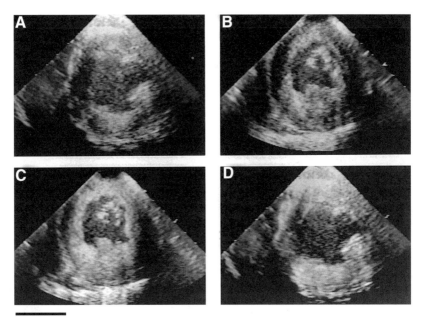

FIGURE 7.

Images of left ventricle short-axis midpapillary muscle level at various stages of contrast injection scored as normal in all regions. **A,** Baseline, just as contrast is beginning to appear in the myocardium. **B,** A few frames later. **C,** A few frames later. **D,** A few frames later. Note: Although a single frame may not appear to completely capture the opacification of all the myocardial regions at once, the temporal filling nature of blood flow into the entire myocardium is captured in multiple frames. (Courtesy of Aronson S, Savage R, Toledano A, et al: Identifying the cause of left ventricular dysfunction after coronary artery bypass graft surgery: The role of myocardial contrast echocardiography. *J Cardiothorac Vasc Anesth* 12:512-518, 1998.)

times those of patients with abnormal flow at 1 week and 18.5 times those of patients with abnormal flow at 1 month. Also in that study, three groups of patients were defined in accordance to their flow-function relationship: (1) patients with normal flow and normal function immediately after separation from bypass (0-60 minutes), as well as normal function at 1 month after surgery; (2) those with normal flow and abnormal function immediately after bypass with normal function at 1 month (ie, stunning); and (3) patients with abnormal flow and abnormal function immediately after bypass and abnormal function at 1 month (ie, old infarction). When the above definitions for flow and function were used, 8% of the myocardial regions were considered stunned at the time immediately after separation from CPB (Figs 8 and 9).

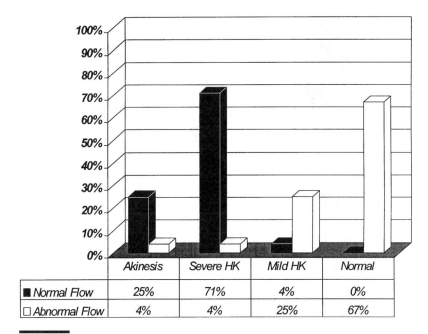

	Akinesis	Severe HK	Mild HK	Normal
■ Normal Flow	25%	71%	4%	0%
□ Abnormal Flow	4%	4%	25%	67%

FIGURE 8.
Bar graph demonstrating flow scores and regional wall motion 12 to 24 hours after separation from cardiopulmonary bypass. Note: 8% of patients had regional flow patterns scored as normal during coronary revascularization (at the time of contrast injection) and subsequent abnormal wall motion in matching regions after separation of cardiopulmonary bypass. *Abbreviation: HK,* Hyperkinesis. (Courtesy of Aronson S, Savage R, Toledano A, et al: Identifying the cause of left ventricular dysfunction after coronary artery bypass graft surgery: The role of myocardial contrast echocardiography. *J Cardiothorac Vasc Anesth* 12:512-518, 1998.)

Assessment of Cardioplegic Solution Perfusion

The infusion of cold potassium cardioplegia solution has been instrumental in reducing the morbidity and mortality associated with open-heart surgery. Optimal myocardial protection during CPB is predicated on adequate homogeneous distribution of cardioplegia solution to all myocardial segments. Traditionally, the efficacy of cardioplegia perfusion has been assessed by quiescence of electrical activity on the ECG, a decrease in myocardial temperature, and direct visualization. Recently, contrast ultrasonography has been used to indicate the adequacy of cardioplegia distribution within the myocardium during cardiac surgery.[92-100]

Monitoring cardioplegia delivery with contrast ultrasound is a direct, real-time, intraoperative technique that enables the surgeon and anesthesiologist to assess the adequacy of cardioplegia distribution to all myocardial segments. Zaroff et al[94] retrospectively investigated the relationship between immediate outcome after cardiac surgery, preoperative LV ejection fraction, and homogeneous delivery of cardioplegia with intraoperative contrast echocardiography in 21 patients undergoing CABG surgery. They found that low ejection fraction alone did not predict low-output failure after CPB, whereas the combination of inadequate intraoperative myocardial protection (as indicated by nonhomogeneous delivery of cardioplegia to myocardial regions at risk) and low ejection fraction always predicted the need for exogenous support to separate from CPB.

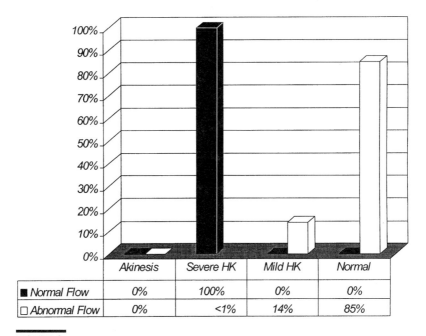

	Akinesis	Severe HK	Mild HK	Normal
■ Normal Flow	0%	100%	0%	0%
□ Abnormal Flow	0%	<1%	14%	85%

FIGURE 9.
Bar graph demonstrating flow scores and regional wall motion at 1 month after coronary artery bypass graft (CABG) surgery. Note: Essentially all segments with flow scores determined to be normal during revascularization while on cardiopulmonary bypass (CPB) are associated with normal regional function at 1 month, and all regions with abnormal flow scores (determined during CABG on CPB) are associated with abnormal regional function at 1 month. *Abbreviation: HK,* Hyperkinesis. (Courtesy of Aronson S, Savage R, Toledano A, et al: Identifying the cause of left ventricular dysfunction after coronary artery bypass graft surgery: The role of myocardial contrast echocardiography. *J Cardiothorac Vasc Anesth* 12:512-518, 1998.)

Although critical coronary artery stenosis may impair antegrade delivery of cardioplegia solutions through the aortic root and thereby contribute to perioperative ischemia and infarction, it has been shown with intraoperative contrast ultrasonography that retrograde infusion of cardioplegia provides myocardial distribution to areas subserved by the left anterior descending and left circumflex coronary arteries even in the presence of complete stenosis of these vessels.[95] Furthermore, retrograde perfusion of cardioplegia (after antegrade cardioplegic induction) in humans has been reported to provide information regarding transmural distribution of cardioplegia, with the ratio of endocardial to epicardial flow being 1.46 ± 0.27 and 1.39 ± 0.33 in the LV free wall and interventricular septum, respectively.[95]

In general, retrograde delivery of cardioplegia for myocardial protection is an approach fostered by coronary venous and arterial anatomy. Its efficacy is highly predicated on individual coronary venous drainage patterns, which vary greatly. Winkelman et al[97] have shown that retrograde delivered cardioplegia through a balloon-tip coronary sinus catheter is not distributed equally to the right ventricle and interventricular septum. They used intraoperative contrast echocardiography and on-line videodensitometric analysis to demonstrate that RV free wall opacification was significantly less (peak pixel intensity, 48 ± 9) compared with the posterior septum (peak pixel intensity, 89 ± 12) or anterior septum (peak pixel intensity, 107 ± 10), after retrograde-delivered cardioplegia.

In a related study by Allen et al,[98] it was confirmed that retrograde cardioplegia provided poor ventricular myocardial perfusion when assessed by contrast echocardiography and coronary ostial drainage. The poor perfusion was unable to meet the myocardial demands of the right ventricle as assessed by oxygen extraction during retrograde perfusion.

Villanueva et al[99] in an experimental protocol used radiolabeled isotopes and MCE to evaluate microvascular flow and nutrient delivery during retrograde and antegrade delivery of cardioplegia. They concluded that microvascular and nutrient flow rates were lower during retrograde delivery because of microvascular differences between coronary arterial and venous systems. Myocardial cooling was, however, equally efficient with either delivery technique, suggesting that the clinical benefits of retrograde delivery primarily resulted from cooling and substrate replenishment and were better achieved (at similar flow rates and temperatures) with antegrade delivery. Their data presumed normal coronary artery anatomy and did not consider the influence of collateralization. In patients with ischemic heart disease, predicting the distribution of cardioplegia and understanding its contribution to myocardial protection in each individual patient is difficult without direct assessment during delivery.

Quintilio et al[100] used intraoperative MCE to determine the myocardial distribution of cardioplegia during combined antegrade and retrograde delivery. They showed that overall myocardial opacification was greater after retrograde delivery in patients with three-vessel disease undergoing elective CABG surgery. However, collateral circulation was the most important determinate for adequacy of myocardial cardioplegia delivery. If adequate collaterals were present, then retrograde delivery offered no advantage for distribution of cardioplegia to regions at risk. On the other hand, they did show that aortic root delivery might not provide adequate myocardial protection in the subset of patients without evidence of significant collateral circulation. MCE remains the only practical method to determine the adequacy of coronary collateral circulation during surgery at the time of cardioplegia delivery.

Assessment of Collateral Myocardial Blood Flow During CABG Surgery

The extent of coronary collateral flow during ischemic heart surgery and its influence on revascularization, myocardial protection, and function recovery have been the focus of many investigators. During coronary bypass surgery, much attention is directed to the coronary angiogram, which provides a roadmap of the degree and location of coronary artery disease. Coronary angiography, however, does not accurately assess the physiologic significance of ischemic heart disease. Angiography remains, nevertheless, the most frequently used technique for assessing collateral blood flow despite only detecting vessels greater than 100 to 200 μm in diameter. Moreover, angiography cannot assess the dynamic functional capacity of collateral vessels. MCE, on the other hand, can be used to demonstrate enhancement in remote regions of the myocardium after intracoronary injections and thereby offer insight into collateral blood flow supplying these regions. The development of coronary artery collateralization that occurs in obstructive coronary artery disease significantly influences distribution of myocardial blood flow and LV function. Spotnitz et al[101] used contrast echocardiography during CABG surgery and reported evidence of collateral flow in six patients. After comparing their results with those predicted with evidence from preoperative coronary angiography, they found that no collateral flow was noted angiographically in three of six patients. Contrast ultrasound techniques (measured background subtracted peak contrast video intensity) demonstrated an increase in collateralization in all six of the patients. In another study by Aronson et al,[102] intraoperative MCE was used during CABG surgery to determine the contribution of collateral blood flow for regional myocardial cardioplegia distribution when delivered antegrade and retrograde. The role of the preoperative ECG and coronary angiogram for determining the distribution of cardioplegia in 15 patients (all with total occlusion of their right coronary artery) was also evaluated and compared with direct assessment with intraoperative MCE. In that study, coronary angiograms were evaluated for native epicardial anatomy and evidence of collateral coronary circulation supplying the right ventricle, LV apex, and interventricular septum. Evaluation of the preoperative ECGs was also performed, and prediction of regional distribution of cardioplegia was compared with delivery of cardioplegia determined with MCE using Albunex. Eighty-seven (97%) of 90 segments were analyzed for cardioplegia distribution at the time of CPB during delivery of cardioplegia. It was demonstrated that the preoperative angiogram and ECG poorly predicted regions at risk for incomplete cardioplegia distribution. Antegrade delivery of cardioplegia was distributed to the right ventricle in 31% of patients despite 100% occlusion of the right coronary artery, whereas retrograde delivery of cardioplegia to the right ventricle only occurred 20% of the time. It was concluded that in the presence of 100% occlusion of the right coronary artery, retrograde cardioplegia delivery is not often observed and antegrade delivery of cardioplegia to the right ventricle is not expected unless coronary collateral circulation is well developed. Furthermore, compared with intraoperative contrast echocardiography, the preoperative angiogram and ECG were not predictive of coronary collateral circulation and therefore not predictive of cardioplegia distribution to the right ventricle.

In conclusion, the application of MCE in the operating room continues to evolve along with the technology itself. There remains much to learn about how to best apply these techniques and the data derived from their use with respect to tailoring therapeutic decisions and clinical pathways. The process, no doubt, will take time and questions about the use of revascularization techniques, myocardial protection strategies, and outcomes will be raised. The opportunity to ask these questions and understand their answers with application of contrast echocardiography holds great promise.

REFERENCES

1. Cheung AT, Savino JS, Weiss SJ, et al: Echocardiographic and hemo-dynamic indexes of left ventricular preload in patients with normal and abnormal ventricular function. *Anesthesiology* 81:376-387, 1994.
2. Reich DL, Konstadt SN, Nejat M, et al: Intraoperative transesophageal echocardiography for the detection of cardiac preload changes induced by transfusion and phlebotomy in pediatric patients. *Anesthesiology* 79:10-15, 1993.
3. Keucherer HF, Muhiudeen IA, Kusumoto FM, et al: Estimation of mean left atrial pressure from transesophageal pulsed Doppler echocardiography of pulmonary venous flow. *Circulation* 82:1127-1139, 1990.
4. Harpole DH, Clements FM, Quill T, et al: Right and left ventricular performance during and after abdominal aortic aneurysm repair. *Ann Surg* 209:356-362, 1989.
5. Gorcsan J III, Gasior TA, Mandarino WA, et al: Assessment of the immediate effects of cardiopulmonary bypass on left ventricular per-formance by on-line pressure-area relations. *Circulation* 89:180-190, 1994.
6. Dell'Italia LJ, Starling MR, Blumhardt R, et al: Comparative effects of volume loading, dobutamine, and nitroprusside in patients with pre-dominant right ventricular infarction. *Circulation* 72:1327-1335, 1985.
7. Vitanen A, Salmenpera M, Heinonen S: Right ventricular response to hypercarbia after cardiac surgery. *Anesthesiology* 73:393-400, 1990.
8. Reichert CL, Visser CA, Koolen JJ, et al: Transesophageal echocardio-graphy in hypotensive patients after cardiac operations: Comparison with hemodynamic parameters. *J Thorac Cardiovasc Surg* 104:321-326, 1992.
9. Rakowski H, Appleton C, Chan KL, et al: Canadian consensus recom-mendations for the measurement and reporting of diastolic dysfunc-tion by echocardiography: From the Investigators of Consensus on Diastolic Dysfunction by Echocardiography. *J Am Soc Echocardiogr* 9:736-760, 1996.
10. Tennant R, Wiggers CJ: The effect of coronary occlusion on myocar-dial infarction. *Am J Physiol* 112:351-361, 1935.
11. Vatner SF: Correlation between acute reductions in myocardial blood flow and function in conscious dogs. *Circ Res* 47:201-207, 1980.
12. Waters DD, Luz PD, Wyatt HL, et al: Early changes in regional and global left ventricular function induced by graded reductions in regional coronary perfusion. *Am J Cardiol* 39:537-543, 1977.
13. Hauser AM, Gangadharan V, Ramos RG, et al: Sequence of mechani-cal, electrocardiographic and clinical effects of repeated coronary artery occlusion in human beings: Echocardiographic observations during coronary angioplasty. *J Am Coll Cardiol* 5:193-197, 1985.
14. Massie BM, Botvinick EH, Brundage BH, et al: Relationship to region-al myocardial perfusion to segmental wall motion: A physiological

basis for understanding the presence of reversibility of asynergy. *Circulation* 58:1154-1163, 1978.

15. Alam M, Khaja F, Brymer J, et al: Echocardiographic evaluation of left ventricular function during coronary angioplasty. *Am J Cardiol* 57:20-25, 1986.

16. Labovitz AJ, Lewen MK, Kern M, et al: Evaluation of left ventricular systolic and diastolic dysfunction during transient myocardial ischemia produced by angioplasty. *J Am Coll Cardiol* 10:748-755, 1988.

17. Pandian NG, Kerber RE: Two-dimensional echocardiography in experimental coronary stenosis: I. Sensitivity and specificity in detecting transient myocardial dyskinesis: Comparison with sonomicrometers. *Circulation* 66:597-602, 1982.

18. Battler A, Froelicher VF, Gallagher KT, et al: Dissociation between regional myocardial dysfunction and ECG changes during ischemia in the conscious dog. *Circulation* 62:735-744, 1980.

19. Tomoike H, Franklin D, Ross J Jr: Detection of myocardial ischemia by regional dysfunction during and after rapid pacing in conscious dogs. *Circulation* 58:48-56, 1978.

20. Smith JS, Cahalan MK, Benefiel DJ, et al: Intraoperative detection of myocardial ischemia in high-risk patients: Electrocardiography versus two-dimensional transesophageal echocardiography. *Circulation* 72:1015-1021, 1985.

21. Wohlgelernter D, Jaffe CC, Cabin HS, et al: Silent ischemia during coronary occlusion produced by balloon inflation: Relation to regional myocardial dysfunction. *J Am Coll Cardiol* 10:491-498, 1987.

22. van Daele ME, Sutherland GR, Mitchell MM, et al: Do changes in pulmonary capillary wedge pressure adequately reflect myocardial ischemia during anesthesia? A correlative preoperative hemodynamic, electrocardiographic, and transesophageal echocardiographic study. *Circulation* 81:865-871, 1990.

23. Leung JM, O'Kelley BF, Browner WS, et al: Prognostic importance of postbypass regional wall-motion abnormalities in patients undergoing coronary artery bypass graft surgery. *Anesthesiology* 71:16-25, 1989.

24. Leung JM, O'Kelley BF, Mangano DT: Relationship of regional wall motion abnormalities to hemodynamic indicies of myocardial oxygen supply and demand on patients undergoing CABG surgery. *Anesthesiology* 73:802-814, 1990.

25. Clements FM, de Bruijn NP: Perioperative evaluation of regional wall motion by transesophageal two-dimensional echocardiography. *Anesth Analg* 66:249-261, 1987.

26. Rosenthal A, Kawasuji M, Takemura H, et al: Transesophageal echocardiography monitoring during coronary artery bypass surgery. *Jpn Circ J* 55:109-116, 1991.

27. Lehmann KG, Forrester AL, McKenzie WB, et al: Onset of altered interventricular septal motion during cardiac surgery. *Circulation* 82:1325-1334, 1990.

28. Chung F, Seyone C, Rakowski H: Transesophageal echocardiography may fail to diagnose perioperative myocardial infarction. *Can J Anaesth* 38:98-101, 1991.

29. Pandian NG, Skorton DJ, Collins SM, et al: Heterogeneity of left ventricular segmental wall motion thickening and excursion in 2-dimensional echocardiograms of normal human subjects. *Am J Cardiol* 51:1667-1673, 1983.

30. Lieberman AN, Weiss JL, Jugdutt BI, et al: Two-dimensional echocardiography and infarct size: Relationship of regional wall motion and thickening to the extent of myocardial infarction in the dog. *Circulation* 63:739-746, 1981.

31. Lima JA, Becker LC, Melin JA, et al: Impaired thickening of nonischemic myocardium during acute regional ischemia in the dog. *Circulation* 71:1048-1059, 1985.

32. Force T, Kemper A, Perkins L, et al: Overestimation of infarct size by quantitative two-dimensional echocardiography: The role of tethering and of analytic procedures. *Circulation* 73:1360-1368, 1986.

33. Braunwald E, Kloner RA: The stunned myocardium: Prolonged, postischemic ventricular dysfunction. *Circulation* 66:1146-1149, 1982.

34. Buffington CW, Coyle RJ: Altered load dependence of postischemic myocardium. *Anesthesiology* 75:464-474, 1991.

35. London MJ, Tubau JF, Wong MG, et al: The "natural history" of in patients undergoing noncardiac surgery. *Anesthesiology* 73:644-655, 1990.

36. Roizen MF, Beaupre PN, Alpert RA, et al: Monitoring with two-dimensional transesophageal echocardiography: Comparison of myocardial function in patients undergoing supraceliac, suprarenal-infraceliac, or infrarenal aortic occlusion. *J Vasc Surg* 2:300-305, 1984.

37. Smith JS, Roizen MF, Cahalan MK, et al: Does anesthetic technique make a difference? Augmentation of systolic blood pressure during carotid endarderectomy: Effects of phenylephrine versus light anesthesia and of isoflurane versus halothane on the incidence of myocardial ischemia. *Anesthesiology* 69:846-853, 1988.

38. Gewertz BL, Kremser PC, Zarins CK, et al: Transesophageal echocardiographic monitoring of myocardial ischemia during vascular surgery. *J Vasc Surg* 5:607-613, 1987.

39. Koenig K, Kasper W, Hofman T, et al: Transesophageal echocardiography for diagnosis of rupture of the ventricular septum or left ventricular papillary muscle during acute myocardial infarction. *Am J Cardiol* 59:362, 1987.

40. Patel AM, Miller FA, Khandheria BK, et al: Role of transesophageal echocardiography in the diagnosis of papillary muscle rupture secondary to myocardial infarction. *Am Heart J* 118:1330-1333, 1989.

41. Gaither NS, Rogan KM, Stajduhar K, et al: Anomalous origin and course of coronary arteries in adults: Identification and improved

imaging utilizing transesophageal echocardiography. *Am Heart J* 122:69-75, 1991.

42. Topol EJ, Humphrey LS, Borkon MA, et al: Value of intraoperative left ventricular microbubbles detected by transesophageal two-dimensional echocardiography in predicting neurologic outcome after cardiac operations. *Am J Cardiol* 56:773- 775, 1985.

43. Oka Y, Inone T, Hong Y, et al: Retained intracardiac air: Transesophageal echocardiography for definition of incidence and monitoring removal by improved techniques. *J Thorac Cardiovasc Surg* 91:329-338, 1986.

44. Topol EJ, Weiss JL, Guzman PA, et al: Immediate improvement of dysfunctional myocardial segments after coronary revascularization: Detection by intraoperative transesophageal echocardiography. *J Am Coll Cardiol* 4:1123-1134, 1984.

45. Koolen JJ, Visser CA, van Wezel HB, et al: Influence of coronary artery bypass surgery on regional left ventricular wall motion: An intraoperative two-dimensional transesophageal echocardiographic study. *J Cardiothorac Vasc Anesth* 1:276-283, 1987.

46. Voci P, Billotta F, Aronson S, et al: Changes in myocardial segmental wall motion, systolic wall thickening, and ejection fraction immediately following CABG: An echocardiographic analysis comparing dysfunctional and normal myocardium. *J Am Soc Echocardiogr* 4:289, 1991.

47. Rahimtoola SH: The hibernating myocardium. *Am Heart J* 117:211-221, 1989.

48. Gould KL: Does positron emission tomography improve patient selection for coronary revascularization? *J Am Coll Cardiol* 20:566-568, 1992.

49. Bolli R: Myocardial 'stunning' in man. *Circulation* 86:1671-1691, 1992.

50. van den Berg EK Jr, Popma JJ, Dehmer GJ, et al: Reversible segmental left ventricular dysfunction after coronary angioplasty. *Circulation* 81:1210-1216, 1990.

51. Marwick TH, Mehta R, Arheart K, et al: Use of exercise echocardiography for prognosis evaluation of patients with known or suspected coronary artery disease. *J Am Coll Cardiol* 30:83-90, 1997.

52. Cigarroa CG, de Filippi CR, Brickner ME, et al: Dobutamine stress echocardiography identifies hibernating myocardium and predicts recovery of left ventricular function after coronary revascularization. *Circulation* 88:430-436, 1993.

53. Nagueh SF, Vaduganathan P, Ali N, et al: Identification of hibernating myocardium: Comparative accuracy of myocardial contrast echocardiography, rest-redistribution thallium-201 tomography and dobutamine echocardiography. *J Am Coll Cardiol* 29:985-993, 1997.

54. Alderman EL, Fisher LD, Litwin P, et al: Results of coronary artery surgery in patient with poor ventricular function. *Circulation* 68:785-795, 1983.

55. Passamani E, Davis KB, Gillespie MJ, et al: A randomized trial of coronary artery bypass surgery: Survival of patients with a low ejection fraction. *N Engl J Med* 312:1665-1671, 1985.

56. Lualdi JC, Douglas PS: Echocardiography for the assessment of myocardial viability. *J Am Soc Echocardiogr* 10:772-780, 1997.

57. Brundage BH, Massie BM, Botvinick EH: Improved regional ventricular function after surgical revascularization. *J Am Coll Cardiol* 3:902-908, 1984.

58. Davila-Roman VG, Waggoner AD, Sicard GA, et al: Dobutamine stress echocardiography predicts surgical outcome in patients with an aortic aneurysm and peripheral vascular disease. *J Am Coll Cardiol* 21:957-963, 1993.

59. Langan EM III, Youkey JR, Franklin DP, et al: Dobutamine stress echocardiography for cardiac risk assessment before aortic surgery. *J Vasc Surg* 18:905-911, 1993.

60. Poldermans D, Fioretti PM, Foster T, et al: Dobutamine-atropine stress echocardiography for assessment of perioperative and late cardiac risk in patients undergoing major vascular surgery. *Eur J Vasc Surg* 8:286-293, 1994.

61. Takeuchi M, Araki M, Nakashima Y, et al: Comparison of dobutamine stress echocardiography and stress thallium-201 single-photon emission computed tomography for detecting coronary artery disease. *J Am Soc Echocardiogr* 6:593-602, 1993.

62. Madu EC, Ahmar W, Arthur J, et al: Clinical utility of digital dobutamine stress echocardiography in the noninvasive evaluation of coronary artery disease. *Arch Intern Med* 154:1065-1072, 1994.

63. Smart SC, Sawada S, Ryan T, et al: Low-dose dobutamine echocardiography detects reversible dysfunction after thrombolytic therapy of acute myocardial infarction. *Circulation* 88:405-415, 1993.

64. Afridi I, Kleiman NS, Raizner AE, et al: Dobutamine echocardiography in myocardial hibernation: Optimal dose and accuracy in predicting recovery of ventricular function after coronary angioplasty. *Circulation* 91:663-670, 1995.

65. Marcovitz PA, Armstrong WF: Dobutamine stress echocardiography: Diagnostic utility. *Herz* 16:372-378, 1991.

66. Senior R, Lahiri A: Enhanced detection of myocardial ischemia by stress dobutamine echocardiography utilizing the "biphasic" response of wall thickening during low and high dose dobutamine infusion. *J Am Coll Cardiol* 26:26-32, 1995.

67. Schiller NB, Shah PM, Crawford M, et al: Recommendations for quantitation of the left ventricle by two-dimensional echocardiography. *J Am Soc Echocardiogr* 2:358, 1989.

68. Martin TW, Seaworth JF, Johns JP, et al: Comparison of adenosine, dipyridamole, and dobutamine in stress echocardiography. *Ann Intern Med* 116:190-196, 1992.

69. Berthe C, Pierard LA, Hiernaux M, et al: Predicting the extent and location of coronary artery disease in acute myocardial infarction by

echocardiography during dobutamine infusion. *Am J Cardiol* 58:1167-1172, 1986.

70. Seeberger MD, Cahalan MK, Chus E, et al: Rapid atrial pacing for detecting provokable demand ischemia in anesthetized patients. *Anesth Analg* 84:1180-1185, 1997.

71. Eichelberger JP, Schwarz KQ, Black ER, et al: Predictive value of dobutamine echocardiography just before non-cardiac vascular surgery. *Am J Cardiol* 72:602-607, 1993.

72. Kiat H, Berman DS, Maddahi J, et al: Late reversibility of tomographic myocardial thallium-201 defects: An acute marker of myocardial viability. *Circulation* 76:1456-1463, 1988.

73. Barilla F, Gheorghiade M, Alam M, et al: Low-dose dobutamine in patients with acute myocardial infarction identifies viable but not contractile myocardium and predicts the magnitude of improvement in wall motion abnormalities in response to coronary revascularization. *Am Heart J* 122:1522-1531, 1991.

74. Voci P, Bilotta F, Caretta Q, et al: Low dose dobutamine echocardiography predicts the early response of dysfunctional myocardial segments to coronary artery bypass grafting. *Am Heart J* 129:521-526, 1995.

75. Di Carli MF, Davidson M, Little R, et al: Value of metabolic imaging with positron emission tomography for evaluating prognosis in patients with coronary artery disease and left ventricular dysfunction. *Am J Cardiol* 73:527-533, 1994.

76. Lee KS, Marwick TH, Cook SA, et al: Prognosis of patients with left ventricular dysfunction, with and without viable myocardium after myocardial infarction: Relative efficacy of medical therapy and revascularization. *Circulation* 90:2687-2694, 1994.

77. Hiratzka LF, McPherson DD, Lamberth WC Jr, et al: Intraoperative evaluation of coronary artery bypass graft anastomosis with high-frequency epicardial echocardiography: Experimental validation and initial patient studies. *Circulation* 73:1199-1205, 1986.

78. Marcus ML, Wilson RF, White CW: Methods of measurement of myocardial blood flow in patients: A critical review. *Circulation* 76:245-253, 1987.

79. Kabas JS, Kisslo J, Flick CL, et al: Intraoperative perfusion contrast echocardiography: Initial experience during coronary artery bypass grafting. *J Thorac Cardiovasc Surg* 99:536-542, 1990.

80. Spotnitz WD, Kaul S: Intraoperative assessment of myocardial perfusion using contrast echocardiography. *Echocardiography* 7:209-228, 1990.

81. Aronson S, Lee BK, Wiencek JG, et al: Assessment of myocardial perfusion during CABG surgery with two-dimensional transesophageal contrast echocardiography. *Anesthesiology* 75:433-440, 1991.

82. Villanueva FS, Spotnitz WD, Jayaweera AR, et al: On-line intraoperative quantitation of regional myocardial perfusion during coronary artery bypass graft operations with myocardial contrast two-dimensional echocardiography. *J Thorac Cardiovasc Surg* 104:1524-1531, 1992.

83. Mudra H, Klauss V, Kreuzer E, et al: Intraoperative assessment of myocardial perfusion before and after bypass grafting by myocardial contrast echocardiography. *Eur Heart J* 13:233, 1992.

84. Aronson S, Savage R, Fernandez A, et al: Assessing myocardial perfusion with Albunex during coronary artery bypass surgery: Technical considerations and safety of aortic root injections. *J Cardiothorac Vasc Anesth* 10:713-718, 1996.

85. Jacobsohn E, Aronson S, Young CJ, et al: On-line contrast echocardiographic assessment of myocardial perfusion: Its role in minimally invasive coronary artery bypass procedures. *J Cardiothorac Vasc Anesth* 11:517-521, 1997.

86. Spotnitz WD, Keller MW, Watson DD, et al: Success of internal mammary bypass grafting can be assessed intraoperatively using myocardial contrast echocardiography. *J Am Coll Cardiol* 12:196-201, 1988.

87. Hirata N, Nakano S, Taniguchi K, et al: Assessment of regional and transmural myocardial perfusion by means of intraoperative myocardial contrast echocardiography during coronary artery bypass grafting. *J Thorac Cardiovasc Surg* 104:1158-1166, 1992.

88. Sabia PJ, Power ER, Ragosta M, et al: An association between collateral blood flow and myocardial viability in patients with recent myocardial infarction. *N Engl J Med* 327:1825-1831, 1992.

89. Ito H, Tomooka T, Sakai N, et al: Lack of myocardial perfusion immediately after successful thrombolysis: A predictor of poor recovery of left ventricular function in anterior myocardial infarction. *Circulation* 85:1699-1705, 1992.

90. Iliceto S, Galiuto L, Marchese A, et al: Analysis of microvascular integrity, contractile reserve, and myocardial viability after acute myocardial infarction by dobutamine echocardiography and myocardial contrast echocardiography. *Am J Cardiol* 77:441-445, 1996.

91. Aronson S, Savage R, Toledano A, et al: Identifying the cause of left ventricular dysfunction after coronary artery bypass graft surgery: The role of myocardial contrast echocardiography. *J Cardiothorac Vasc Anesth* 12:512-518, 1998.

92. Villanueva FS, Kaul S, Glasheen WP, et al: Intraoperative assessment of the distribution of retrograde cardioplegia using myocardial contrast echocardiography. *Surg Forum* 12:252-254, 1990.

93. Voci P, Bilotta F, Caretta Q, et al: Mechanisms of incomplete cardioplegia distribution during coronary artery surgery: An intraoperative transesophageal contrast echocardiography study. *Anesthesiology* 79:904-912, 1993.

94. Zaroff J, Aronson S, Lee BK, et al: The relationship between immediate outcome after cardiac surgery, homogeneous cardioplegia delivery, and ejection fraction. *Chest* 106:38-45, 1994.

95. Aronson S, Lee BK, Zaroff JG, et al: Myocardial distribution of cardioplegic solution after retrograde delivery in patients undergoing cardiac surgical procedures. *J Thorac Cardiovasc Surg* 105:214-221, 1993.

96. Aronson S, Lee BK, Liddicoat JR, et al: Assessment of retrograde cardioplegia distribution using contrast echocardiography. *Ann Thorac Surg* 52:810-814, 1991.

97. Winkelmann J, Aronson S, Young CJ, et al: Retrograde-delivered cardioplegia is not equally distributed to the right ventricle free wall and septum. *J Cardiothorac Vasc Anesth* 9:135-139, 1995.

98. Allen BS, Winkelmann JW, Hanafy H, et al: Retrograde cardioplegia does not adequately perfuse the right ventricle. *J Thorac Cardiovasc Surg* 109:1116-1126, 1995.

99. Villanueva FS, Spotnitz WD, Glasheen WP, et al: New insights into the physiology of retrograde cardioplegia delivery. *Am J Physiol* 268:H1555-H1566, 1995.

100. Quintilio C, Voci P, Bilotta F, et al: Risk factors of incomplete cardioplegic solution during coronary artery grafting. *J Thorac Cardiovasc Surg* 109:439-447, 1995.

101. Spotnitz WD, Matthew TL, Keller MW, et al: Intraoperative demonstration of coronary collateral flow using myocardial contrast two-dimensional echocardiography. *Am J Cardiol* 65:1259-1261, 1990.

102. Aronson S, Jacobsohn E, Savage R, et al: The influence of collateral flow on the antegrade and retrograde distribution of cardioplegia in patients with an occluded right coronary artery. *Anesthesiology* 89:246-254, 1998.

CHAPTER 8

Uncommon Coagulation Problems

Jan Charles Horrow, MD
Clinical Professor, Anesthesiology, MCP Hahnemann University,
Philadelphia; Vice President, Clinical Development, IBEX Technologies
Corporation, Malvern, Pennsylvania

Patients who are about to undergo cardiac surgery may have an uncommon coagulation disorder that has been previously diagnosed, or they may have an unusual coagulation problem that arises during the perioperative period. This chapter will address selected topics of both types, with the latter type discussed first.

HEPARIN-INDUCED THROMBOCYTOPENIA
CASE PRESENTATION
A 44-year-old woman entered the hospital after 8 months of progressive clinical deterioration after viral myocarditis and subsequent cardiomyopathy. After 6 weeks' therapy, including increasing doses of dobutamine as well as other cardiotonic and antidysrhythmic agents, she underwent placement of a left ventricular assist device. She received heparin for that procedure and a heparin infusion after it. Subsequent daily platelet counts were 160, 162, 140, 145, 90, 75, and 45×10^9/L, respectively. Her physicians discontinued heparin therapy on the fifth postoperative day and commenced warfarin therapy. She now awaits heart transplantation.

PATHOPHYSIOLOGY
Platelets secrete platelet factor 4 (PF4), which combines with heparin in their vicinity, forming complexes that occasionally engender antibody formation. These immunoglobulin G antibodies combine with specific receptors (FcγII) on the platelet surface, activating them. Activation releases PF4, further fueling this phenomenon (Fig 1).

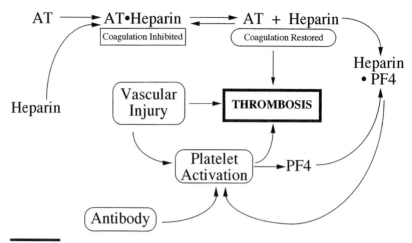

FIGURE 1.
Events leading to heparin-induced thrombosis. First, heparin and antithrombin *(AT)* form a complex *(AT•heparin)*. Platelet activation, resulting from antibody to heparin•PF4 complexes, releases PF4, which binds heparin, driving the dissociation reaction for AT•heparin to the right. This restores coagulation locally, leading to thrombus formation on injured endothelium. (Courtesy of Parmet JL, Horrow JC: Hematologic diseases, in Benumof JL [ed]: *Anesthesia and Uncommon Diseases*, ed 4. Philadelphia, WB Saunders, 1998, p 296.)

Platelets, activated by this process, are removed from circulation, thus decreasing the platelet count. Less commonly, damaged endothelium forms a site for platelet adhesion, forming thrombi that obstruct vessels and result in organ damage. Thrombosis occurs despite heparin presence because the PF4 secreted from platelet activation serves not only to form more antigenic complexes but also to neutralize the heparin nearby.

DIFFERENTIAL DIAGNOSIS
Heparin predictably decreases platelet count. Because not all decreases in platelet count are antibody mediated, we classify heparin-induced thrombocytopenia (HIT) as type I (predictable, mild decreases accompanying heparin therapy) or type II (more severe, antibody-mediated decreases with or without accompanying thrombosis).

In type II HIT, the platelet count decreases within 2 weeks (median, 10 days) of the start of heparin therapy to between 20 and 150×10^9/L. Normal platelet counts in a patient who had previously exhibited a thrombocytosis also suggest type II HIT. The pattern matters, rather than absolute numbers.

Confirmatory diagnosis requires either a serotonin release assay performed with patient's plasma and donor platelets or an enzyme-linked immunosorbent assay (ELISA) that detects antibodies to the heparin-PF4 complex. The tests must use the type and formulation of heparin administered to the patient because of the wide variability of heparin preparations.

PREVALENCE

Most data on prevalence are limited by their incompleteness or questionable confirmatory tests. Prevalence increases with duration of exposure to heparin: about 1% after 7 days' infusion, and 3% after 14 days. Bovine heparin may engender HIT more frequently (5.5%) than porcine heparin (1%), although this distinction requires better data to achieve more widespread acceptance.

The upper bound of the incidence of HIT with thrombosis after 5 days of heparin therapy is about 1%. This statistic generates great concern because of the frequent use of heparin infusions and the high likelihood that HIT with thrombosis can progress to loss of life or limb.

TREATMENT

All exposure to heparin must cease immediately. This includes heparin-bonded catheters, heparin flush solutions, and pressure-monitoring tubing with slow infusions of dilute heparin. Also, low–molecular weight heparin should be witheld, unless it has been specifically tested and known to be nonimmunogenic.

An alternative method of anticoagulation should be substituted, unless the risks of anticoagulation cessation are small. Few options exist in many surgical scenarios: all are experimental or beyond approved labeling. Table 1 lists these options.

For the patient requiring cardiopulmonary bypass, the two most viable options are the dermatan-heparin combination agent danaparoid (Orgaran) or the direct thrombin inhibitor hirudin. Both agents are currently marketed in the United States, although for different indications. Unfortunately, a neutralizing agent does not exist for either agent.

COLD AGGLUTININS
PATHOPHYSIOLOGY

Some patients harbor autoantibodies which, after structural changes induced by cold, agglutinate red blood cells. These patients present in one of three ways: they may carry this diagnosis; routine laboratory testing may discover this disorder; or the

TABLE 1.

Treatment Alternatives for Anticoagulating Patients With HIT for Bypass

Alternative	Mechanism	Disadvantages
Delay surgery, then heparin	Antibodies regress	Surgery often cannot wait
Ancrod	Destroys fibrinogen	Long preparation time Not easily reversed
Plasmapheresis, then heparin	Removes antibody	Long preparation time May not remove all antibody
Low–molecular weight heparin	Inhibits factor Xa	Antibodies may cross-react Dose for bypass unknown No point-of-care monitor Protamine neutralizes poorly
Iloprost, then heparin	Platelet inhibition	Not available in United States Extreme vasodilation
Danaparoid (mixture of dermatan and low–molecular weight heparin)	Dermatan inhibits heparin cofactor II	Dose for bypass unknown No point-of-care monitor No reversal agent
Lepirudin (recombinant hirudin); Argatroban	Direct thrombin inhibitors	No reversal agent

Abbreviation: HIT, Heparin-induced thrombocytopenia.

operating surgeon may observe the agglutinated red blood cells during hypothermic bypass.

In the first instance, the threshold temperature for agglutination may also be known. Most often, the threshold falls below moderate levels of hypothermia (32°C). If discovered during preoperative screening, the hospital clinical laboratory measures the threshold so that physicians will know the safe limits of hypothermia. Some centers routinely test for cold agglutinins. The laboratory will communicate the temperature threshold and titer for such newly diagnosed cases. Higher temperatures and higher titers imply more difficult management.

PREPARATION FOR SURGERY

When known in advance, the simplest strategy maintains perfusion temperature above the agglutinin threshold. Occasionally hypothermia is unavoidable—for example, when using deep hypothermic circulatory arrest. Preoperative plasmapheresis, which removes the offending antibody and decreases titers markedly, permits safe conduct of bypass at hypothermia. Consultation with a blood bank specialist can optimize this process.

CONDUCT OF BYPASS

Unfortunately, the most common presentation occurs during bypass when, much to the consternation of the operating surgeon, as the patient cools, innumerable red clumps begin to polka-dot the surgical field. Surgical loops accentuate this bizarre appearance. In this case, increasing perfusion temperature will usually halt the process. Surgeons should undertake whatever modifications are necessary to ensure myocardial preservation. The blood bank can use existing or new clot to perform cold agglutinins testing so that the actual titer and temperature threshold can be determined as soon as possible. If ignored, hemolysis, renal failure, and myocardial damage might ensue.

HEPARIN RESISTANCE

CASE PRESENTATION

A 64-year-old 100-kg man arrives from the catheterization laborary with an intra-aortic balloon in place for aortocoronary bypass grafting. He receives intravenous infusions of nitroglycerin and heparin. Table 2 chronicles physicians' attempts to achieve their target activated clotting time (ACT) of 480 seconds to institute bypass. After administering 650 units/kg, the physicians ordered fresh frozen plasma, which is given when it arrives later. In the meantime, they administer additional heparin, which achieves the ACT threshold, allowing bypass to commence at 1700 hours.

How should clinicians approach neutralization of heparin after termination of bypass?

PATHOPHYSIOLOGY

Concentrations of the coagulation factors that are considerably less than half of normal still permit full physiologic function of fibrinogen formation. However, when concentrations of the coagulation inhibitors, antithrombin among them, decrease to as little as 75% of normal, thrombotic disorders may manifest. Chronic infusions of heparin decrease circulating concentrations of

TABLE 2.

Attempted Anticoagulation in Heparin
Resistance

Time*	Heparin (units)	ACT (sec)
1500	—	145
1600	40,000	382
1613	10,000	447
1635	15,000	438
1700	15,000	510
1720	—	493
1740	2 units FFP	—
1745	Cool to 28°C	>1000
1820	—	903

*Times are military wall clock values.
Abbreviations: ACT, Activated clotting time; *FFP,* fresh
frozen plasma.

antithrombin, the endogenous substance responsible for heparin's inhibition of thrombin. Nitroglycerin infusions may compound this effect. Both kaolin and celite ACTs decrease substantially in antithrombin-deficient blood. For example, blood containing 2.5 units/mL heparin normally has a 450-second celite ACT. This decreases to 320 seconds when antithrombin concentration halves.

DIFFERENTIAL DIAGNOSIS

Inadequate prolongation of the ACT might also arise from a defective device. For this and other reasons, such devices undergo quality control checks several times each day. Because heparin is a biological product with variable activity, some physicians also switch to another type, brand, or lot of heparin before labeling a patient as heparin resistant. Increases in concentrations of coagulation factor VIII alone will decrease the ACT response to heparin administration; doubling factor VIII concentration reduces an ACT of 425 seconds to approximately 360 seconds.

MANAGEMENT

Although some clinicians believe that it is heparin concentration and not ACT that matters in establishing anticoagulation for bypass, most agree that this approach courts disaster by ignoring the pharmacodynamic aspects of drug action. Management strategies include administration of larger doses of heparin, antithrombin concentrate, or fresh frozen plasma. The last choice potentially exposes the patient to blood-borne pathogens. Antithrombin concentrate, labeled for treatment of sepsis rather than for antithrombin deficiency, does not transmit infectious agents. It has not yet achieved widespread availability. For the case presented, physicians administered fresh frozen plasma once it became available. Whether because of fresh frozen plasma, hypothermic bypass, or their combination, the resultant ACT overshot the target by exceeding 1000 seconds.

The author attains acceptable ACT values in such cases by administering additional doses of heparin. This strategy uses hypothermic bypass, an upper limit of 1000 units/kg total heparin, and a slightly lower threshold for acceptable ACT values (ie, 425 instead of 480 seconds). Because these patients will require additional protamine for neutralization, particular attention to slow infusion of protamine is important to minimize the adverse responses to protamine. For the case presented, 420 mg of protamine returned the ACT to only 260 seconds. Another 100 mg reduced it further to 190 seconds. Finally, a third dose of protamine, this one 50 mg, yielded an ACT of 150 seconds.

ALLERGY TO PROTAMINE
CASE PRESENTATION
An 86-year-old man has received NPH insulin for 10 years to treat diabetes mellitus. Three years ago he underwent multivessel coronary artery bypass grafting. At that time, at the conclusion of a 10-minute infusion of 300 mg of protamine, his systemic blood pressure suddenly decreased from 130/74 to 78/38 mm Hg, and pulmonary arterial pressure decreased from 34/19 to 14/6 mm Hg. Hemodynamics stabilized after administration of 2 L clear fluid, 1 L albumin, 3 units packed red blood cells, diphenhydramine 50 mg, methylprednisolone 1 g, and epinephrine 100 μg push followed by an infusion of 16 μ/min for 3 hours. After a prolonged postoperative course, he was discharged and returned to his usual activities.

PATHOPHYSIOLOGY
Three types of adverse responses to protamine occur. Type I is characterized by a predictable decrease in systemic blood pressure after rapid (<3 minutes) intravenous administration. Release of histamine or other vasoactive substances from mast cells mediates this response. In type II reactions, antibodies to

protamine result in capillary leak, causing bronchospasm, edema, decreased filling pressures, and substantial systemic and pulmonary arterial hypotension. Histamine and other mediators of anaphylaxis mediate this response. In type III reactions, heparin-protamine complexes release thromboxane from the lung, resulting in marked increases in pulmonary artery pressure, right heart failure, and resultant systemic hypotension. Increased pulmonary pressure may also result from polycation-induced inhibition of nitric oxide synthase. Protamine also causes platelet dysfunction, inhibits thrombin at high concentrations, and may be associated with perioperative myocardial infarction.

Several factors increase the risk of an adverse protamine reaction. Previous long-term exposure to protamine-containing insulin preparations increases this risk by several orders of magnitude. Patients allergic to true fish may possess antibodies that cross-react with antigenic determinants on protamine, a substance derived from the crushed gonads of male salmon. Likewise, vasectomy increases the likelihood of presence of anti-sperm antibodies that cross-react with protamine antigenic determinants. Patients with chronic pulmonary hypertension from valvular or other causes may manifest type III responses more commonly.

DIFFERENTIAL DIAGNOSIS

This chapter will not attempt to list the various causes of systemic hypotension during cardiac surgery. Vasodilation and mechanical maneuvers are the most obvious confounding influences. Halting protamine administration may help differentiate the cause. Return of both systemic and pulmonary pressures to the normal range within a few minutes suggests a type I or type III protamine reaction. Confirmation of protamine allergy (type II) remains elusive, however, because a readily available ELISA does not exist and skin tests display poor specificity.

MANAGEMENT

Table 3 presents options in managing patients with known protamine allergy. Allowing heparin's effects to dissipate naturally commits physicians to the administration of large amounts of allogeneic blood products and exposes the patient to the risks of blood-borne infection, hypovolemia, hypotension, and consumptive coagulopathy. Currently, no commercially available alternative to protamine exists.

TABLE 3.
Alternatives to Protamine for Neutralization of Unfractionated Heparin

Alternative	Mechanism	Disadvantages
Allow heparin effect to dissipate	Metabolism/excretion	Massive hemorrhage Massive transfusion requirement
Hexadimethrine	Polyanion-polycation	Toxicity similar to protamine Renal toxicity also
Methylene blue	Anion-cation	Does not decrease ACT Pulmonary hypertension
Platelet transfusions	Polyanion-polycation	Does not decrease ACT Massive transfusion requirement
Platelet factor 4	Polyanion-polycation	Not available in United States May not avoid adverse responses
Heparinase I	Enzymatically degrades heparin	Investigational drug Residual anti-Xa activity (benefit?)
Designer polycations	Polyanion-polycation	Investigational drugs May retain toxicity of protamine
Lactoferrin	Polyanion-polycation	Investigational drug ACT not completely normalized
Protamine filter in pump	Polyanion-polycation	Investigational device Risks coagulation during process

Abbreviation: ACT, Activated clotting time.

FACTOR DEFICIENCIES: HEMOPHILIAS
PATHOPHYSIOLOGY

Genes coding for coagulation factors VIII and IX reside on the X chromosome, leading to sex-linked transmission; female carriers transmit the defective gene to half of their sons. In hemophilia A, factor VIII is synthesized but is defective. Patients with hemophilia B may or may not possess factor IX antigenic material. Deficiency of either factor impairs activation of factor X (Fig 2),

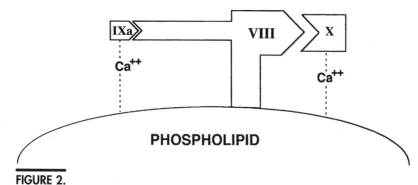

FIGURE 2.
Activation of factor X requires both factors VIII and IX, the former acting as cofactor in the activation sequence. Patients with hemophilia A lack functioning factor VIII. Those with hemophilia B lack sufficient factor IX. (Courtesy of Horrow JC: Desmopressin and antifibrinolytics. *Int Anesthesiol Clin* 28[4]:230-236, 1990.)

prolonging the activated partial thromboplastin time. The bleeding time, which reflects platelet function, remains normal. Hemophilia varies in severity; mild cases possess more than 5% normal factor coagulant activity, moderate ones between 1% and 5% activity, and severe cases less than 1% activity. The overall prevalence is 2 per 10,000 males. Patients who are about to undergo cardiac surgery would rarely have undiagnosed hemophilia.

PREPARATION FOR SURGERY
Surgical hemostasis requires at least 80% of factor VIII or 60% of factor IX coagulant activity, with at least 30% factor VIII or 20% factor IX activity until postoperative day 10. Desmopressin, 0.3 µg/kg, increases factor VIII coagulant activity twofold to fourfold by releasing large multimers of von Willebrand factor from endothelium. Patients with mild or moderate hemophilia A may require only desmopressin to prepare for surgery. However, a trial several days before surgery to confirm sufficient response must occur because individual response to desmopressin varies. Processed blood products can supply additional factor VIII if needed. These include cryoprecipitate, factor VIII concentrate, recombinant products, and fresh frozen plasma.

Patients with hemophilia B obtain factor IX replacement from factor IX concentrate, recombinant products, or fresh frozen plasma. Because the half-life of factor IX in the body is nearly triple that of factor VIII but its bioavailability is only half that of factor VIII, calculation of the dosing scheme for factor IX replacement differs substantially from that of factor VIII. Consultation with a qualified hematologist will guide management of initial and continuing postoperative factor replacement therapy.

After replacement of the missing factor and arrangements for postoperative replacement, surgery may proceed without other modifications. Replacement almost always precedes incision, rather than occurring on termination of bypass. Additional factor replacement may be given on bypass to account for hemodilution, taking into account that the normal response of an increase in factor VIII activity during bypass may not occur in patients with hemophilia A.

FACTOR DEFICIENCIES: VON WILLEBRAND DISEASE
CASE PRESENTATION
A 45-year-old woman is seen for replacement of her rheumatic mitral valve. She wears a Medi-Alert bracelet that reads "von Willebrand disease." She describes "nearly bleeding to death" after cosmetic surgery 5 years ago. However, she underwent three uneventful vaginal deliveries. Her symptoms include frequent nosebleeds and heavy menses.

PATHOPHYSIOLOGY
Endothelium secretes von Willebrand factor, which then binds to it and to marginating platelets to mediate platelet adhesion. Von Willebrand factor also protects circulating factor VIII from degradation and facilitates its secretion.

The expected prevalence of von Willebrand disease is 1.4 to 5 cases per 1000 population, making it the most common inherited coagualation disorder. In classic von Willebrand disease (type I, 70%-80%), von Willebrand factor multimers are normal but present in decreased amounts. Abnormal multimers occur in type II von Willebrand disease (13%-17%). In type III (1%-3%), synthesis of von Willebrand factor is totally absent.

Because von Willebrand factor is an acute-phase reactant, its concentrations vary widely. Oral contraceptives, infection, pregnancy, surgery, and other stresses increase von Willebrand factor concentration, confounding diagnostic efforts. Unlike hemophiliacs, patients with von Willebrand disease who are about to undergo surgery may not have had von Willebrand disease previously diagnosed. A medical history focusing on bleeding events may raise suspicions. This is also one instance in which a preoperative bleeding time will prove worthwhile. Decreased ristocetin cofactor activity confirms diagnosis. Innumoelectrophoresis can typify and quantitate the extent of disease.

PREPARATION FOR SURGERY

Desmopressin, 0.3 µg/kg administered intravenously over 20 to 30 minutes, constitutes the treatment of choice for patients with mild or moderate type I von Willebrand disease. It will triple or quadruple plasma concentrations of von Willebrand factor. For other types of von Willebrand disease, desmopressin is either ineffective or will precipitate thrombocytopenia. A trial several days before elective surgery should confirm adequate response before depending on this therapeutic option. Fresh frozen plasma, cryoprecipitate, and commercial concentrates provide additional von Willebrand factor replacement. As with hemophiliacs, patients with von Willebrand disease will benefit from the perioperative recommendations of a qualified hematologist.

Surgery should proceed in the usual fashion after securing arrangements to establish and maintain suitable von Willebrand factor plasma activity. Surgical hemostasis requires between 80% and 100% activity, which should be maintained after hemodilution on bypass.

RARE FACTOR DEFICIENCIES

Nearly all other factor deficiencies (prothrombin, fibrinogen, V, VII, X, XI, XIII) display autosomal recessive inheritance. Intraoperative diagnosis of these rare inherited disorders is extraordinarily unlikely. For a patient who has such a diagnosis, consultation with a qualified hematologist should include providing the consultant with information regarding the changes wrought by bypass on coagulation factors (Fig 3), so that suitable augmentation may occur on termination of bypass. Bleeding after cardiac surgery in factor-deficient patients may arise from failure to account for hemodilution on bypass.

SICKLE CELL DISEASE
CASE PRESENTATION

A 32-year-old woman with hemoglobin SS disease requires mitral valve replacement for insufficiency. She has atrial fibrillation, congestive heart failure, asthma, and chronic renal insufficiency (serum creatinine, 1.8 mg/dL). Medications include digoxin and inhaled steroids. Her hemoglobin concentration is 7.2 g/dL, of which 85% is hemoglobin S.

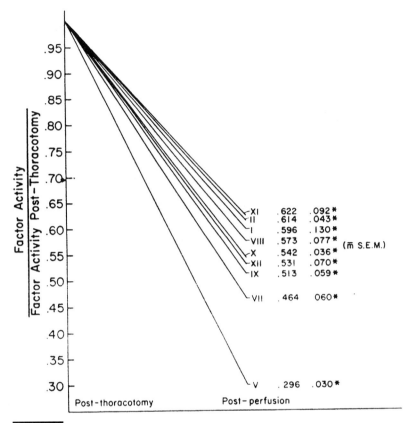

FIGURE 3.
Fraction of coagulation factor activity on institution of bypass, reflecting the effect of hemodilution. (Courtesy of Kalter RD, Saul CM, Wetstein L, et al: Cardiopulmonary bypass: Associated hemostatic abnormalities. *J Thorac Cardiovasc Surg* 77:427-435, 1979.)

PATHOPHYSIOLOGY

Hemoglobin S, compared with normal hemoglobin, is 50-fold less soluble in the desaturated state, forming stacks of molecules that deform the cell membrane into a sickled shape. Patients have multiple systemic effects from bouts of sickling, including thrombotic or hemorrhagic cerebral infarction, cardiomegaly, increased pulmonary vascular resistance with right heart failure, ventilation-perfusion mismatch, splenic sequestration of red blood cells and platelets, pigmented cholelithiasis, renal papillary necrosis, and aseptic femoral necrosis.

PREPARATION FOR SURGERY

Decreasing the total amount of hemoglobin S will permit hypothermic bypass. Methods to achieve this decrease vary substantially; Table 4 lists them. All involve removal of red blood cells containing the defective hemoglobin and replacement with normal banked homologous red blood cells. Replacement of hemoglobin S with hemoglobin A may require more than a dozen units of packed red blood cells, depending on the patient's blood volume and hydration status. This exchange may occur days or hours before surgery, during operation, or at the beginning of bypass.

CONDUCT OF BYPASS

To avoid sickle crises, the environment of all tissue capillary beds should be maintained to avoid stasis, low oxygen tension, and decreased pH. Ample intravenous hydration before bypass, hemodilution during bypass, enriched oxygen mixtures to the lungs and the pump oxygenator, and frequent arterial pH determination with aggressive bicarbonate therapy contribute to these goals. Complete warming during bypass will facilitate maintenance of normothermia in the immediate postoperative period.

SICKLE CELL TRAIT

Patients with sickle cell trait make both hemoglobin A and S. They do not exhibit the end-organ damage seen in those homozygous for

TABLE 4.

Methods to Decrease Hemoglobin S Concentration

Method	Timing	Disadvantages
Simple transfusion	Several weeks before surgery	Elective cases only Volume overload
Partial exchange transfusion before operation	Day(s) before surgery	Elective cases only Large volume shifts Multiple donor exposures
Exchange transfusion with cell separation	Day of surgery	Large volume shifts Multiple donor exposures
Intraoperative exchange transfusion ± cell separation	At start of bypass	Multiple donor exposures

the disease. However, the extremely acidic and concentrated environment of the renal medulla promotes sickling, so that by adulthood infarction has occurred in the renal medulla of patients with sickle cell trait causing isosthenuria. Although several reports demonstrate that such patients tolerate hypothermic bypass without sequelae, many physicians prefer to perform a limited exchange transfusion before instituting hypothermia. This management strategy should consider the risks of allogeneic blood exposure.

RECENT ANTIPLATELET THERAPY
PHARMACOLOGY

Surgeons have dealt with the hemostatic sequelae of recent aspirin ingestion for at least a decade. However, our cardiology colleagues continue to embrace new therapeutic options in the catheterization laboratory that have an impact on the care of patients who require urgent surgery after an interventional cardiology procedure. This section will consider the challenge presented by use of platelet glycoprotein inhibitors.

Abciximab (Reopro), a fragment of a human-murine monoclonal antibody, binds irreversibly to platelet glycoprotein receptor IIb/IIIa, thus blocking platelet aggregation. Its rapid half-life in plasma (10 minutes), resulting from prompt binding to circulating platelets, belies its nearly 48-hour duration of action. Platelet binding can last for the duration of the platelet life span.

Eptifibitide (Integrelin), a cyclic peptide RGD antagonist, and tirofiban (Aggrastat) and its congeners, which are nonpeptide mimetics, bind reversibly to the active site of the glycoprotein IIb/IIIa receptor.

PERIOPERATIVE MANAGEMENT

Only platelet transfusions can offset the effects of abciximab. However, platelet-bound drug equilibrates rapidly with newly transfused platelets, inhibiting them. Physicians must administer sufficient platelets to overwhelm the drug present. Untreated, the bleeding time returns to less than 12 minutes within 24 hours in 90% of patients.

The short half-lives of eptifibitide and tirofiban, 2.5 and 2 hours, respectively, permit some recovery of platelet function in patients who require bypass surgery. Nevertheless, for patients undergoing heparin neutralization after bypass within 5 hours of drug exposure, transfusion of platelets should occur early in the event of poor hemostasis.

SUGGESTED READING

Agarwal SK, Ghosh PK, Gupta D: Cardiac surgery and cold-reactive proteins. *Ann Thorac Surg* 60:1143-1150, 1995.

Balasundaram MS, Duran CG, al-Halees Z, et al: Cardiopulmonary bypass in sickle cell anemia: Report of five cases. *J Cardiovasc Surg* 32:271-274, 1991.

Brieger DB, Mak KH, Kottke-Marchant K, et al: Heparin-induced thrombocytopenia. *J Am Coll Cardiol* 31:1449-1459, 1998.

Despotis GJ, Levine V, Heinrish JJ, et al: Antithrombin III during cardiac surgery: Effect of response of activated clotting time to heparin and relationship to markers of hemostatic activation. *Anesth Analg* 85:498-506, 1997.

Horrow JC: Protamine: A review of its toxicity. *Anesth Analg* 64:348-361, 1985.

Lusher JM: Congenital coagulopathies and their management, in Rossi EC, Simon TL, Moss GS, et al (eds): *Principles of Transfusion Medicine*, ed 2. Baltimore, Md, Williams & Wilkins, 1996, pp 423-452.

Madan M, Berkowitz SD, Tcheng JE: Glycoprotein IIb/IIIa integrin blockade. *Circulation* 98:2629-2635, 1998.

Parmet JL, Horrow JC: Hematologic diseases, in Benumof JL (ed): *Anesthesia and Uncommon Diseases*, ed 4. Philadelphia, WB Saunders, 1998, pp 274-315.

Phillips DR, Scarborough RM: Clinical pharmacology of eptifibatide. *Am J Cardiol* 80:11B-20B, 1997.

Warkentin TE, Hayward CPM, Boshkov LK, et al: Sera from patients with heparin-induced thrombocytopenia generate platelet-derived microparticles with procoagulant activity: An explanation for the thrombotic complications of heparin-induced thrombocytopenia. *Blood* 84:3691, 1994.

C HAPTER 9

How to Construct a Monocusp Valve

Steven R. Gundry, MD
Professor and Head, Division of Cardiothoracic Surgery, Loma Linda
University Medical Center, Loma Linda, California

T he surgical relief of obstructions of the right ventricular outflow tract and pulmonary annulus by both closed and open
techniques produced some of the earliest success stories in congenital cardiac surgery.[1-3] However, when relief of the obstruction
is accompanied by gross pulmonary insufficiency, the physiologic
changes that occur can result in significant hemodynamic compromise. This compromise may be especially severe when relief of
obstructions accompany intracardiac repair, as was demonstrated
by Ellison and others in the 1950s.[4-7] As these sequelae became
manifest, concern for the morbidity after a transannular patch has
convinced many surgeons that leaving an imperfect and stenotic
native pulmonary valve is preferable to acute and long-term pulmonary insufficiency. Although possibly adequate in both the
short term and long term, continued disappointment with this
strategy has prompted the application of other methods for restoring right ventricle to pulmonary artery continuity, using valved
conduits, homografts, or monocusp valves in concert with a
transannular patch. The methods and materials used in construction of a monocusp are legion, and often of such complexity that it
has remained a little used tool, despite its well-described clinical
utility. Because our group first began using a pulmonary monocusp in 1972, we have amassed a considerable experience, which
in turn has resulted in a simplified construction and application of
the pulmonary monocusp valve.[8] The details of its construction
and application are described in this chapter.

MONOCUSP CONSTRUCTION

After traditional right ventriculotomy, pulmonary arteriotomy, or both, the need for pulmonary annular enlargement is assessed by any number of surgical judgment tools or formulas. If pulmonary valve stenosis is accompanied by right ventricular outflow tract muscular obstruction, infundibular resection is carried out, followed by pulmonary valvectomy. The level of the pulmonary annulus is identified, and a choice of monocusp material is made (Fig 1). In general, autologous pericardium has been the material of choice for both the monocusp and the transannular patch in newborns and infants. However, in older children, in whom previous operations may have depleted the supply of native pericardium, or who have significant pulmonary artery distortion that may predict later pulmonary artery hypertension, we have used Gortex surgical membrane (Gore, Inc, Flagstaff, Ariz) or bovine pericardium to construct the monocusp and transannular patch.

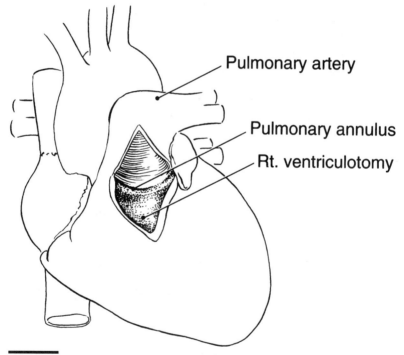

Pulmonary artery

Pulmonary annulus

Rt. ventriculotomy

FIGURE 1.

Right ventriculotomy and pulmonary arteriotomy in right ventricular outflow tract reconstruction. (Courtesy of Gundry SR: Pericardial and synthetic monocusp valves. *Semin Thorac Cardiovasc Surg* 2:77-82, 1999.)

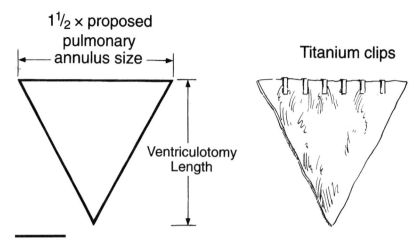

FIGURE 2.
Left, Approximate proportions and measurements for the monocusp valve, which is constructed of autologous or bovine pericardium or Gortex pericardial membrane. **Right,** Titanium clips are utilized on the free edge of the monocusp to provide weight and to facilitate a to-and-fro motion of the valve. (Courtesy of Gundry SR: Pericardial and synthetic monocusp valves. *Semin Thorac Cardiovasc Surg* 2:77-82, 1999.)

Indeed, studies just reported from our laboratory, using a growing sheep model, have suggested that a Gortex monocusp combined with a Gortex transannular patch may provide long-term monocusp function.[9]

The material to be used for the monocusp is cut in a roughly triangular shape with the base of the triangle measuring approximately 1.5 times the proposed pulmonary annular size, with the height of the triangle being approximately the length of the ventriculotomy (Fig 2). In actual practice, we cut the monocusp to be more generous than the actual measurements because we can always trim extra length as the implantation proceeds. Moreover, if a Gortex monocusp is used in a growing child, it should be oversized to prevent late stenosis. After trimming of the monocusp, titanium surgical clips are attached to the free edge of the valve, small clips for infants and medium clips for older children. These five to six clips are designed to mimic the natural increased weight at the edge of the normal human valve so that inertia is created, resulting in closure of the valve during diastole.

Next, the monocusp valve is draped into the right ventriculotomy, with the leading edge aligned with the level of the proposed pulmonary valve annulus. We have used two equally effective techniques for attaching the monocusp to the ventriculotomy. The approach we began with proceeds immediately to sew the edges of the monocusp to the right ventricular outflow tract ventriculotomy walls using running monofilament sutures. This is followed by attachment of the transannular patch over the monocusp/right ventricular suture line, followed by or preceded by attaching the transannular patch onto the edges of the pulmonary arteriotomy. Although perfectly acceptable, this technique results in a double and unnecessary suture line. Currently, our preferred technique is to sew both the monocusp and the transannular patch to the right ventriculotomy simultaneously, as illustrated in Figure 3. In general, the distal tip of the transannular patch is sewn to the pulmonary arteriotomy and brought toward the pulmonary annulus. When this point is reached, both the monocusp edge and the transannular patch are sewn as a single suture line (with the

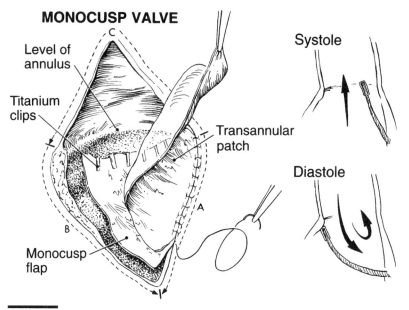

FIGURE 3.
Left, The sequential suturing of the monocusp flap and transannular patch as a single step in transannular patching of the right ventricular outflow tract. The monocusp flap and the transannular patch can also be sewn individually to the edges of the right ventriculotomy. **Right,** The position of the valve open in systole and closed in diastole. (Courtesy of Gundry SR: Pericardial and synthetic monocusp valves. *Semin Thorac Cardiovasc Surg* 2:77-82, 1999.)

monocusp "sandwiched" between the right ventriclular muscle and the transannular patch). This is illustrated by suture lines *A* and *B* in Figure 3. The surgeon, of course, can use any combination of sewing order (ie, *A, B,* then *C*) to complete the transannular patch and monocusp insertion.

Our laboratory studies have suggested that the best long-term function of the monocusp is achieved using Gortex surgical membrane as the monocusp coupled with a transannular patch of Gortex. Nevertheless, we rarely use this combination clinically because persistent bleeding may occur. The Gortex transannular patch can be covered with autologous or bovine pericardium to reduce this tendency. Because the laboratory studies are so compelling, it is likely that we will use more of the double Gortex combination in the future, keeping in mind that the Gortex must be oversized to allow for growth when used in young children and infants.

Function of the monocusp can usually be ascertained in the operating room by visually seeing the monocusp move beneath the autologous pericardial patch once blood flow is reestablished. However, when not visible, a closing click can be felt when palpating the transannular patch. Finally, transesophageal or handheld echocardiography can be used to detect monocusp motion, as illustrated in Figure 3.

SUMMARY

Construction of a monocusp is an easy procedure that adds little, if any time to routine transannular patching of the right ventricular outflow tract. It also adds little cost to the operation when constructed from autologous pericardium. The monocusp's utility in preventing or lessening the impact of pulmonary regurgitation in the early postoperative period has been demonstrated. Its utility as a long-term pulmonary valve substitute will need to await longer-term clinical follow-up currently underway at our institution and others.

REFERENCES

1. Fuster V, McGoom DC, Kennedy MA, et al: Long-term evaluation (12 to 22 years) of open heart surgery for tetralogy of Fallot. *Am J Cardiol* 46:635-642, 1980.
2. Kirklin JW, Ellis HF Jr, McGoom DC, et al: Surgical treatment for the tetralogy of Fallot by open intra-cardiac repair. *J Thorac Cardiovasc Surg* 37:22-48, 1959.
3. Poirier RA, McGoom DC, Danielson GK: Late results after repair of tetralogy of Fallot. *J Thorac Cardiovasc Surg* 73:900-909, 1977.
4. Ellison RG, Brown WJ Jr, Hague EE Jr, et al: Physiologic observations in experimental pulmonary insufficiency. *J Thorac Surg* 30:633-641, 1955.

5. Ellison RG, Brown WJ Jr, Yeh TJ, et al: Surgical significance of acute and chronic pulmonary valvular insufficiency. *J Thorac Cardiovasc Surg* 60:549-558, 1970.

6. Bender HW, Austen WG, Ebert PA, et al: Experimental pulmonic regurgitation. *J Thorac Cardiovasc Surg* 45:451-459, 1963.

7. Austen WG, Greenfield LJ, Ebert PA, et al: Experimental study of right ventricular function after surgical procedures involving the right ventricle and pulmonic valve. *Ann Surg* 155:606-613, 1962.

8. Gundry SR, Razzouk AJ, Boskind JF, et al: Fate of the pericardial monocusp pulmonary valve for right ventricular outflow tract reconstruction: Early function, late failure without obstruction. *J Thorac Cardiovasc Surgery* 107:908-913, 1994.

9. Izutani H, Gundry SR, Vricella LA, et al: Right ventricular outflow tract reconstruction using Gore-Tex membrane monocusp valve in infant animal. *ASAIO J*, in press.

CHAPTER 10

Extracardiac Conduit Variation of the Fontan Procedure

Ed Petrossian, MD
Assistant Professor of Surgery, University of California, San Francisco;
Pediatric Cardiothoracic Surgeon, Valley Children's Hospital, Madera,
California

LeNardo D. Thompson, MD
Associate Professor of Surgery, University of California, San Francisco;
Pediatric Cardiothoracic Surgeon, Oakland Children's Hospital, Oakland,
California

Frank L. Hanley, MD
Professor of Surgery and Pediatric Cardiothoracic Surgeon, University of
California, San Francisco

Despite steady advances in surgical technique, patients who undergo a Fontan operation continue to be at increased risk for short- and long-term morbidity and mortality. Follow-up studies have shown that most of the morbidity and mortality is related to ventricular failure, arrhythmias, and consequences of elevated systemic venous pressure.[1-4] To optimize outcome after the Fontan operation, it is therefore important to preserve ventricular function, avoid arrhythmias, and undertake measures to reduce systemic venous pressure including preservation of pulmonary vascular function and construction of a Fontan pathway with laminar flow dynamics. Among the modifications of the Fontan operation currently used, the extracardiac conduit approach may offer the greatest potential for achieving these goals and optimizing postoperative outcome.

Since 1992, at the University of California, San Francisco (UCSF), we have used the extracardiac conduit Fontan (ECF) as the procedure of choice for palliation of patients with functional single ventricle physiology. In this chapter, we describe the evolution of our approach to the ECF operation.

FONTAN PHYSIOLOGY

Because of lack of a pulmonary ventricle, patients who undergo a Fontan operation have marginal hemodynamics. Small disturbances in ventricular or pulmonary vascular function, turbulent flow in the Fontan circuit, or atrial dysrhythmias translate into elevated systemic venous (Fontan) pressure and poor outcome. This is best appreciated by highlighting the circulatory physiology of a Fontan connection. As depicted in Figure 1, the Fontan circulation is an in-series circulation in which a single power source (the ventricle) is used to propel blood through a series of two resistance units (the systemic and pulmonary vascular beds). Blood is conducted through these components via three series of vascular conduits. The increased pressure work of two resistance units in series puts the ventricle at risk for systolic and diastolic dysfunction. In addition, the absence of a pulmonary ventricle forces the conduit connecting the two resistors (the systemic veins, the Fontan connection, and the pulmonary arteries in series) to conduct blood at pressures sufficient

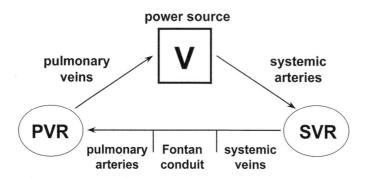

FIGURE 1.
Schematic representation of Fontan circulation, demonstrating the in-series configuration. The single ventricle *(V)* is the only power source for moving blood through the two resistance components, the systemic vascular resistance *(SVR)* and pulmonary vascular resistance *(PVR)*. Conducting blood between the power source and the two resistors are three conduits: the systemic arteries, a combination of systemic veins–Fontan connection–pulmonary arteries, and the pulmonary veins. (Courtesy of Petrossian E, McElhinney DB, Reddy VM, et al: The role of the extracardiac conduit as a cavopulmonary anastomosis in the evolution of the Fontan procedure, in Redington AN, Deanfield JE, Brawn WJ, et al [eds]: *The Right Heart in Congenital Heart Disease.* London, Greenwich Media Limited, 1998, pp 149-156.)

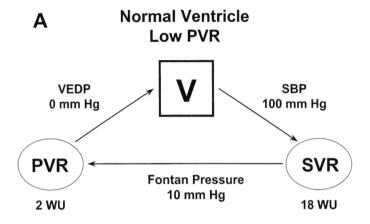

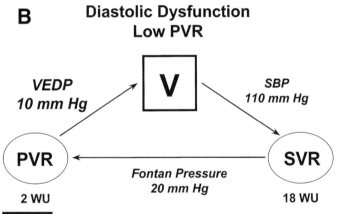

FIGURE 2.
Illustration of the adverse effects of diastolic dysfunction and elevated pulmonary vascular resistance *(PVR)* on Fontan hemodynamics. **A,** With normal ventricular function and PVR, the pressure in the Fontan connection may be estimated at 10 mm Hg. **B,** With ventricular dysfunction, the ventricular end-diastolic pressure *(VEDP)* rises to 10 mm Hg, which translates into an increase in the Fontan pressure to 20 mm Hg.

(continued)

to overcome pulmonary vascular resistance (Fig 2, A). This results in a delicate balance in which the stability of the entire circulation is sensitive to small changes in its separate components. Small increases in ventricular end-diastolic pressure (Fig 2, B) or pulmonary vascular resistance (Fig 2, C) can lead to significantly increased Fontan pressure and poor outcome. The stability of the circulation therefore

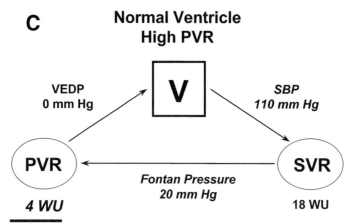

FIGURE 2. (continued)
C, An increase in PVR from 2 to 4 Wood units *(WU)* also translates into a 10 mm Hg increase in Fontan pressure. These calculations are based on an assumed baseline systemic blood pressure *(SBP)* of 100 to 110 mm Hg, systemic vascular resistance *(SVR)* of 18 WU, and a cardiac output of 5 L/min. (Courtesy of Petrossian E, McElhinney DB, Reddy VM, et al: The role of the extracardian conduit as a cavopulmonary anastomosis in the evolution of the Fontan procedure, in Redington AN, Deanfield JE, Brawn WJ, et al [eds]: *The Right Heart in Congenital Heart Disease.* London, Greenwich Media Limited, 1998, pp 149-156.)

requires optimal functioning of each component, including (1) a power source that is able to handle the increased pressure work without systolic or diastolic dysfunction, (2) a Fontan connection that has laminar flow dynamics and extracts minimal energy from the systemic venous circuit, and (3) low resistance in the second resistor (pulmonary vascular bed). One additional factor that is important in optimizing Fontan hemodynamics is preservation of sinus rhythm. For the most part, failure to satisfy one or more of these criteria is responsible for the various complications that can occur early and late after a Fontan operation. In each of these areas, the extracardiac approach may have advantages over other types of Fontan connection, such as the atriopulmonary or lateral tunnel procedures.

EVOLUTION OF THE FONTAN OPERATION

The original Fontan operation was based on the principle that the right atrium could contribute to pulsatile flow in the systemic venous circuit.[5] An important turning point in the evolution of the Fontan operation has been the hydrodynamic studies conducted by de Leval et al[6] showing that improved flows can be obtained in the Fontan circulation by excluding the right atrium from the circuit. The pulsating and irregularly shaped right atrial cavity was shown to generate significant impediments to forward flow, which could be overcome by effectively bypassing the right atrium using a more streamlined tubular pathway. This was accomplished by the lateral tunnel Fontan operation in which the venous return from the inferior vena cava (IVC) is channeled to the pulmonary artery by placement of a baffle against the inside lateral wall of the right atrium.[6-8] The more laminar flow pattern in this pathway functions to lower resistance and preserve kinetic energy, thereby improving forward flow in the systemic venous circuit.

Another important strategy in the evolution of the Fontan operation has been the concept of staged operations with an initial bidirectional Glenn procedure followed by a completion Fontan operation. Before a bidirectional Glenn procedure, because of the underlying parallel circulation, the single ventricle is accustomed to a high-preload, low-afterload physiology. As a result, the ventricular geometry is modeled to do volume work with an enlarged cavity volume and increased myocardial muscle mass. After a primary Fontan operation, without an intervening bidirectional Glenn, the ventricle becomes abruptly exposed to a low-preload, high-afterload physiology. This acute alteration in hemodynamics, brought about by a direct transition from parallel circulation to Fontan circulation, causes unfavorable ventricular geometry by increasing the mass-to-volume ratio.[9] This in turn may lead to compromised diastolic and systolic function and poor outcome.[10] An intervening bidirectional Glenn operation, in conjunction with removal of the parallel circulation, allows for abolishment of the chronic volume overload on the ventricle, at no cost to oxygenation.[11,12] The ventricular geometry is allowed to adapt and remodel in response to the reduced volume work, and become better prepared for the ultimate Fontan physiology. We recommend an early bidirectional Glenn (between 3 and 4 months of age) to preserve ventricular function by minimizing the duration of time that the ventricle is exposed to a volume over-loaded state.[13,14] In addition, an early Glenn operation will help preserve pulmonary vascular function by preventing the development of pulmonary vascular obstructive disease, and avoid pulmonary artery distortion, complications that may occur in patients with prolonged exposure to parallel circulation.

A further advance in the Fontan operation has been the concept of incomplete partitioning of the systemic and pulmonary venous circuits in the form of an adjustable atrial septal defect (ASD) or fenestration of the Fontan circuit.[15-18] During the early postoperative period, ventricular and pulmonary vascular function become transiently depressed because of the well-known negative effects of cardiopulmonary bypass, hypothermia, and ischemic cardiac arrest. Transient alterations in ventricular and pulmonary vascular function lead to poor forward flow through the Fontan circuit. This translates into elevated systemic venous (Fontan) pressure, low preload for the ventricle, and low cardiac output, and may lead to early postoperative death or failure requiring takedown after the Fontan operation.[4,19,20] These complications may occur especially in patients with marginal preoperative hemodynamics or patients who are left with mild residual lesions such as pulmonary artery stenosis or atrioventricular valvar regurgitation. A controlled right-to-left shunt in the form of an adjustable ASD or small fenestration in the Fontan circuit allows for sufficient augmentation of preload for the ventricle so that cardiac output is optimized with resultant improvement of early postoperative outcome.[16-18] Furthermore, simultaneous decompression of the systemic venous circuit allows for lower Fontan pressure and has been shown to decrease the incidence of pleural and pericardial effusions.[4]

With the above significant advances in surgical technique and staging of the operation, outcomes after the modified Fontan operation improved considerably, and several centers reported encouraging results.[3,4,19,21] Despite these advances, however, results after a modified Fontan operation remained less than optimal. Mortality was greatest in the early postoperative period,[4,19] a fact that underscores the importance of perioperative management for the overall success of the Fontan operation. Whereas Fontan fenestration has improved early outcomes after the operation, the price to be paid for creation of a right-to-left shunt includes systemic desaturation, risk of systemic embolization, and the need for an additional procedure for closure of the fenestration. Most importantly, early and late supraventricular arrhythmias continued to be a persistent source of morbidity after the atriopulmonary and lateral tunnel Fontan operations.[22-27]

The ECF operation was originally described by Humes et al[28] and Nawa and Teramoto[29] in 1988. This variation of the Fontan principle was initially applied to heterotaxy patients with anomalies of pulmonary and systemic venous drainage and common atrioventricular valve. In 1990, Marcelletti et al[30] reported the ECF operation in four patients with "(1) hypoplasia or atresia of the left atrioventricular valve, (2) common atrioventricular valve, (3) anomalies of systemic and pulmonary venous return, or (4) auricular juxtaposition." In these reports, the initial impetus for an extracardiac approach was concern about intraatrial obstruction to flow, either at the level of the pulmonary veins or the atrioventric-ular valve, caused by the intraatrial partition used to separate sys-temic and pulmonary venous blood in the traditional atriopul-monary variation of the Fontan operation.[30,31] Marcelletti et al subsequently recognized the hydrodynamic advantages of the ECF operation and its potential for decreasing postoperative atrial tachy-arrhythmias, and they applied this variation of the Fontan opera-tion to all patients with functional single ventricle physiology.[31,32]

THE UCSF EXPERIENCE

At UCSF, we initially became interested in the ECF operation in 1992 because of its potential for improving both perioperative and long-term outcome. At about this time, many groups using the lat-eral tunnel Fontan began to report a disturbing incidence of atrial dysrhythmias[22,23] as well as the need to frequently use an adjustable ASD or fenestration to minimize perioperative morbid-ity.[16,17] Four of the advantages of the ECF operation that we per-ceived as being critical in improving postoperative results include (1) preservation of ventricular function by avoiding aortic cross-clamping; (2) preservation of ventricular and pulmonary vascular function by minimizing cardiopulmonary bypass time and avoid-ing hypothermia; (3) preservation of sinus rhythm by avoiding atrial incisions and suture lines and surgery in the vicinity of the sinus node; and (4) the potential for optimal flow dynamics in the ECF circuit.

NO AORTIC CROSS-CLAMPING

Because of the inherently marginal nature of the Fontan circula-tion, along with the alterations in ventricular mass-to-volume ratio during the transition to a Fontan circulation, it is important to pre-serve ventricular function to optimize postoperative cardiac out-put. Prolonged aortic cross-clamp time has been shown to be asso-ciated with early death or Fontan failure requiring takedown.[20] An important advantage of the extracardiac approach is that because entry into the heart is not required, the operation can be performed on a beating heart and without cross-clamping the aorta. Previously, the procedure, as described by Marcelletti et al,[30] involved deep hypothermia, cardioplegic arrest, and total circula-tory arrest. In our experience, unless an intracardiac procedure was necessary, aortic cross-clamping was altogether avoided. In addition, to prevent the need for an intracardiac procedure at the time of the Fontan operation, we made every effort to perform most ancillary intracardiac procedures (such as atrial septectomy,

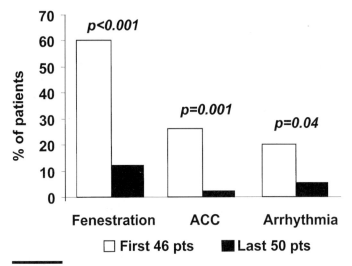

FIGURE 3.
Evolution of the extracardiac conduit Fontan operation at the University of California, San Francisco. Comparison of the first 46 patients with the last 50 patients in the series revealed a significant decrease in the incidence of aortic cross-clamping (*ACC*), atrial tachyarrhythmias, and Fontan pathway fenestration.

valve repair, relief of outflow tract obstruction) at the time of the Glenn operation. This ensures that the procedure at the time of the Fontan operation is limited to placement of the extracardiac conduit alone (along with pulmonary arterioplasty if necessary). Of the 96 patients who underwent a primary (nonrevision) ECF operation at our institution, only 12 patients (13%) required cross-clamping of the aorta. During the course of our experience, we have become more adamant in this respect, which is reflected by the fact that only 1 (2%) of the last 50 patients required aortic cross-clamping compared with 11 (24%) of the first 46 patients (Fig 3).

MINIMAL CARDIOPULMONARY BYPASS TIME
Prolonged cardiopulmonary bypass (CPB) time is associated with increased risk of early postoperative death or failure requiring takedown after the Fontan operation.[4,19] Prolonged hypothermic CPB also has well-known negative sequelae on ventricular and pulmonary vascular function. In our experience, the intraoperative postbypass common atrial pressure, an indirect measure of ventricular diastolic function, was significantly higher in patients

with longer CPB times (Fig 4). The intraoperative postbypass Fontan pressure, a measure of pulmonary vascular function in patients with normal ventricular function, was also significantly higher in patients with prolonged CPB time (Fig 5). Furthermore, patients who required a perioperative fenestration, a marker of cardiopulmonary dysfunction, had significantly longer CPB times compared with patients who did not require a fenestration (Fig 6). These findings lend support to our contention that perioperative ventricular and pulmonary vascular function can be optimized by limiting the duration of CPB.

With increasing experience with the ECF operation, we soon realized that CPB time could be significantly reduced by performing the entire conduit to pulmonary artery anastomosis off bypass. This is accomplished by partial occlusion of the branch pulmonary arteries, allowing the bidirectional Glenn shunt to perfuse one or both lungs while performing the conduit to pulmonary artery anastomosis (Fig 7). With this technique, only partial CPB is needed (IVC venous cannulation only), and the duration of bypass is limited to the time necessary to perform the IVC to conduit anastomosis. To optimize ventricular function, the bypass circuit is primed with blood and supplemented with calcium. Hypothermia

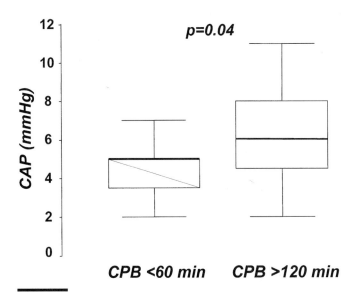

FIGURE 4.
Effect of duration of cardiopulmonary bypass *(CPB)* on common atrial pressure *(CAP)*. Longer bypass times are associated with significantly higher CAPs.

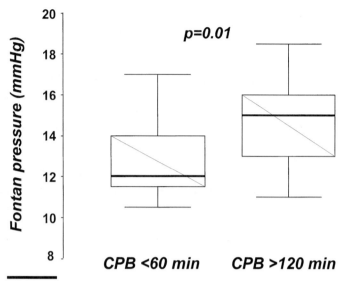

FIGURE 5.
Effect of duration of cardiopulmonary bypass *(CPB)* on Fontan pressure.
Longer bypass times are associated with significantly higher Fontan pressures.

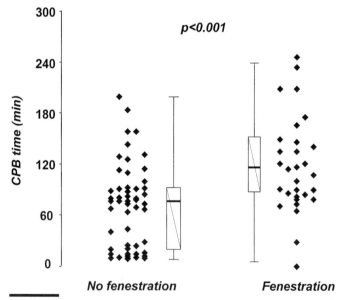

FIGURE 6.
Effect of duration of cardiopulmonary bypass *(CPB)* on fenestration of the
Fontan pathway. Patients who required a perioperative fenestration had
significantly longer CPB times.

A

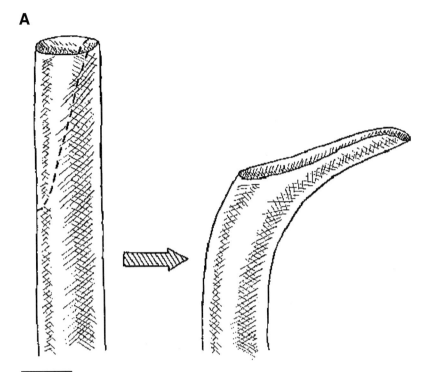

FIGURE 7.
Operative technique for the extracardiac conduit Fontan. **A,** A polytetra-fluoroethylene (PTFE) conduit slightly larger than the inferior vena cava (IVC) diameter is selected and appropriately beveled to allow for a large anastomotic opening and to relieve branch pulmonary artery stenoses.

(continued)

is avoided and the operation is done on a warm beating heart. We started using this technique in 24 of the last 31 patients in the series, and in this group, median partial CPB time was only 12 minutes (range, 9-41 minutes).

At an extreme the ECF operation can be performed entirely off bypass.[33] The IVC to conduit anastomosis is performed by temporarily diverting the IVC flow to the right atrium. We recently have experimented with this technique and believe it represents an acceptable alternative in appropriate candidates.[34]

REDUCTION OF ATRIAL DYSRHYTHMIAS
In our experience, one of the most promising advantages of ECF operation has been its ability to reduce atrial dysrhythmias, which in most centers continues to be a persistent source of morbidity

B

C

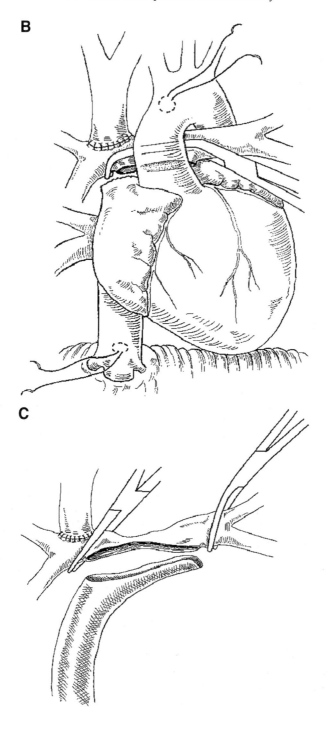

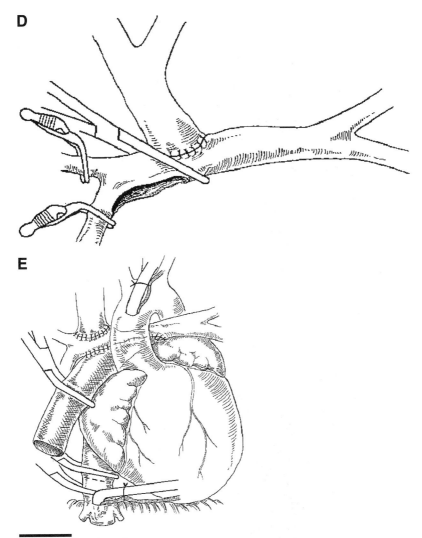

FIGURE 7. (continued)
B-D, The conduit to pulmonary artery anastomosis is performed off bypass using partial occlusion of the branch pulmonary arteries, allowing the bidirectional Glenn shunt to perfuse both lungs **(B)** or either the right **(C)** or the left lung **(D)** depending on the presence and location of branch pulmonary artery stenoses. **E,** The IVC is mobilized to the level of the hepatic veins to make room for the subsequent cannulation and anastomosis. The IVC to conduit anastomosis is performed on partial bypass by cannulating the aorta and IVC alone, and allowing the Glenn to continue to perfuse the lungs.

(continued)

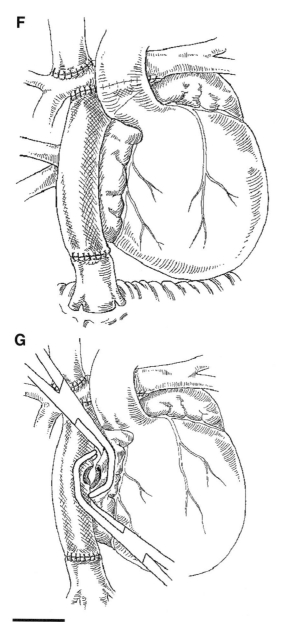

FIGURE 7. (continued)
F, The completed operation. **G,** Construction of a fenestration, off bypass using partial occlusion vascular clamps, either directly using a side-to-side anastomosis, or with the interposition of a small PTFE tube graft.

and mortality after the Fontan operation.[22-27] The ECF operation addresses each of the three primary factors that are important potential contributors to post-Fontan atrial tachyarrhythmias: (1) exposure of the right atrium to the elevated systemic venous pressure with subsequent atrial dilatation, hypertrophy, and fibrosis; (2) extensive atrial incisions and suture lines[25]; and (3) surgery in the vicinity of the sinus node.[26] In the lateral tunnel Fontan operation, a portion of the right atrial wall remains exposed to the elevated systemic venous pressure and is therefore at risk for dilatation, hypertrophy, and fibrosis, causing atrial arrhythmias. In the ECF operation, however, the right atrium is entirely excluded from the high-pressure systemic venous circulation. In addition, an atrial incision and extensive atrial suture lines are an inherent part of the lateral tunnel Fontan operation, whereas the ECF operation is performed with an atrial "no touch" technique in which incisions and suture lines are altogether avoided. Finally, surgery in the vicinity of the sinus node or its vascular supply, as is the case in the hemi-Fontan operation, is also avoided in the ECF operation.

In our series of 96 patients undergoing a primary ECF operation, only 5 patients (5%) had new, transient, early postoperative supraventricular tachyarrhythmias (SVT), including junctional ectopic tachycardia in 4 and atrial flutter in 1. New transient sinus node dysfunction (SND) requiring temporary pacing occurred in 7 patients (7%) in the early postoperative period. On late follow-up, only 2 patients (2%) had recurrent atrial dysrhythmias. It is difficult to separate the influence of prior procedures on the development of these arrhythmias because not all patients in the series of 96 patients received neonatal and subsequent procedures at our institution.

With improvements in our preoperative strategies and intraoperative techniques for preservation of ventricular function that evolved during the course of our experience, we have seen the incidence of early postoperative atrial dysrhythmias decrease significantly among our last 50 patients (Fig 3). In this group, none of the patients had new-onset SVT, and only 2 patients had SND. The figures above compare favorably to the 14% to 32% incidence of atrial dysrhythmias (including SVT and SND) reported recently for the lateral tunnel and atriopulmonary Fontan operations.[3,19,26,27] Although these results are encouraging, long-term follow-up will be necessary to confirm the advantages of the extracardiac approach in decreasing the incidence of late postoperative atrial dysrhythmias.

HEMODYNAMIC EFFICIENCY

The hemodynamic advantages of a tubular Fontan pathway have been demonstrated convincingly by hydrodynamic and computational modeling studies.[6,35,36] The extracardiac Fontan conduit is made of a smoothly contoured circumferential tube, and the right atrium is entirely excluded from the Fontan circuit. This has the advantage of optimizing laminar flow patterns and avoiding the possible future development of turbulence and stasis associated with atrial dilatation, as may be the case for the lateral tunnel Fontan operation. Direct experimental comparison of hydrodynamic efficiency of the three commonly used tubular Fontan pathways, including the traditional intraatrial lateral tunnel, the extracardiac (epicardial) lateral tunnel, and the extracardiac conduit, has shown that the extracardiac conduit variation of the Fontan operation extracts significantly less energy than the two lateral tunnel techniques.[37] The above studies have also demonstrated that technical modifications of the Fontan to pulmonary artery connection can further minimize energy dissipation, and therefore lead to improved long-term outcome by allowing the Fontan circuit to operate at low systemic venous pressures. Energy dissipation is lowered when the Fontan to pulmonary artery connection is made as large as possible.[36] Energy dissipation can be further minimized by displacing (offsetting) the inferior cavopulmonary anastomosis away from that of the superior cavopulmonary anastomosis.[35-37] We have found the extracardiac conduit approach to be ideally suited for achieving the above two technical modifications. The conduit to pulmonary artery anastomosis can be conveniently enlarged as much as necessary by cutting the graft with a generous bevel (Fig 7, A). Using this technique, the pulmonary artery anastomotic opening can be made as much as two times the diameter of the conduit.

The direction of offset is usually determined by the presence and location of branch pulmonary artery stenoses. In the presence of branch pulmonary artery stenoses, the conduit is incorporated into an aggressive pulmonary arterioplasty either medially toward the pulmonary trunk (Fig 7, C) or laterally toward the right lower lobe pulmonary artery (Fig 7, D). This technique allows for simultaneous offsetting of the superior and inferior cavopulmonary anastomoses and relief of branch pulmonary artery stenoses. It has the additional advantage of simplifying the operation by obviating the need for separate patch material for the pulmonary artery reconstruction. An additional advantage of the ECF operation, as compared with the lateral tunnel technique,[36] is that offsetting of the two anastomoses is achieved without the need to operate in the vicinity of the sinus node.

REDUCTION OF FONTAN FENESTRATION

The ability to perform the ECF operation as a "closed" procedure without the need to enter the heart poses a new question regarding the role of routinely leaving an adjustable ASD or fenestration in the Fontan pathway. Improved results have been reported using these maneuvers with the lateral tunnel Fontan operation.[4,16-18] In this setting, the purpose of the fenestration is to optimize Fontan hemodynamics in the early postoperative period. Because most of the patients who undergo the ECF operation require only a short duration of partial bypass and no cardioplegic arrest, their postbypass Fontan hemodynamics may be more favorable than those of patients who require prolonged CPB, hypothermia, and myocardial ischemia.

Instead of routine fenestration, we therefore recommend fenestrating only those patients who demonstrate objective evidence of poor or marginal postpump hemodynamics. This approach is especially suitable with the extracardiac technique because the fenestration can be conveniently performed as a closed procedure without resuming bypass, either in the operating room or, if needed, postoperatively in the intensive care unit (Fig 7, G). By limiting fenestration to those patients who will derive a hemodynamic benefit from a postoperative right-to-left shunt, we hope to avoid the potential morbidities associated with fenestration including systemic desaturation, systemic embolization, and the need for an additional procedure for fenestration closure.

Among 96 consecutive patients undergoing a primary ECF operation at our institution, we fenestrated the extracardiac conduit in only 32 patients (33%). More importantly, the number of patients requiring a fenestration decreased significantly during the course of our experience with only 6 of the last 50 patients (12%) being discharged home with a fenestration (Fig 3). We attribute this decrease in the need for fenestration to several factors that evolved during the course of our experience including a decrease in the incidence of aortic cross-clamping, a decrease in CPB time, avoidance of hypothermia, a decrease in the incidence of atrial dysrhythmias, and improvements in construction of a Fontan circuit with minimal energy dissipation. Of the 24 patients who underwent the ECF operation with minimal CPB time by performing the conduit to PA anastomosis off bypass, only 1 patient (4%) required fenestration.

PLEURAL EFFUSIONS

Pleural and pericardial effusions have been a persistent source of morbidity and delay in hospital discharge in patients undergoing a Fontan operation. In our experience, median duration of chest tube drainage was 8 days, and prolonged drainage (more than 2 weeks) occurred in 19% of the patients. This is similar to the 13% to 39% incidence of prolonged drainage reported recently for other types of Fontan operation.[3,4,17,18,38] Our approach to removing chest tubes in patients who undergo a Fontan operation is extremely conservative. Chest tubes are not removed unless the drainage is less than 1 mL/kg/d for at least 2 days. Although this approach prolongs the duration of time before chest tubes are removed, it functions to decrease the incidence of readmission for recurrent effusions. We recognize the reported role of fenestration in decreasing postoperative effusions[4]; however, because of lack of a control group we cannot draw inferences regarding the need for fenestration based on our effusion data. Our analysis nevertheless has not shown the duration of chest tube drainage to be significantly different between fenestrated and nonfenestrated patients.

GROWTH POTENTIAL

The ECF operation has potential disadvantages that relate to the use of a prosthetic conduit, including lack of growth potential, Fontan pathway obstruction, and thromboembolism. In an effort to incorporate growth potential in the design of the operation, Laschinger et al[39-41] introduced the extracardiac lateral tunnel (ELT) Fontan, which involves placement of an incomplete prosthetic conduit on the epicardial surface of the right atrium to direct IVC flow to the pulmonary arteries. This technique is essentially a mirror image of the lateral tunnel Fontan in which the prosthetic "baffle" is placed on the outer aspect of the right atrium. An advantage of this technique is avoidance of a circumferential conduit and therefore maintenance of radial growth potential in the Fontan connection. Gundry et al[42] subsequently reported a variation of the ELT in which autologous pedicled pericardium is used to construct the epicardial baffle. Although growth potential is theoretically maintained by the ELT operation, a major disadvantage of this technique is that it is potentially arrhythmogenic. The operation requires extensive atrial suture lines, some of which are in close proximity to the sinus node or its vascular supply. Furthermore, the right atrial wall is exposed to the elevated systemic venous pressure and is therefore at risk for dilatation. This may lead to flow turbulence and stasis in the Fontan pathway and also to obstruction at the level of the pulmonary veins or the atrioventricular valve.

In another attempt to incorporate growth potential into the operation, Okabe et al[43] reported a variation of the ECF technique in which the conduit is constructed using autologous pedicled pericardium that is rolled into a tube and sewn to itself with a longitudinal suture line. The suitability of this technique depends on the availability of sufficient amount of pedicled pericardium to construct a nonobstructive circumferential conduit with an adequately large pulmonary anastomotic opening. Although theoretically attractive, this operation may have limited applicability in the setting of a staged operation and a redo sternotomy in which sufficient amount of pericardium may not be available.

Because of the disadvantages of the above techniques, we continue to use a polytetrafluoroethylene (PTFE) conduit to construct the extracardiac Fontan pathway. To address the lack of growth potential in the conduit, we wait until the patient weighs about 15 kg (approximately 3-4 years of age) before performing the procedure. With this strategy, we expect to avoid reoperation by using an adult-sized conduit (20-22 mm), which should accommodate the patient's future growth and exercise demands. By staging the operation with an intervening bidirectional Glenn, with or without an additional source of pulmonary blood flow, significant exercise-induced cyanosis does not usually occur until patients start using more extensive lower-body exercise at about 4 to 5 years of age. The strategy of performing the operation at 3 to 4 years of age, therefore, does not expose the patients to prolonged cyanosis. Furthermore, because the patient's ventricle and pulmonary vasculature have been unloaded with an early bidirectional Glenn, development of ventricular dysfunction or pulmonary vascular obstructive disease is no longer a concern while the patient is waiting to reach Fontan age. We do, however, recommend an early Fontan operation in the unusual event that the patient develops evidence of pulmonary arteriovenous malformations.

FONTAN PATHWAY OBSTRUCTION

Development of pathway obstruction has been described in extracardiac conduits used for the atriopulmonary or atrioventricular variation of the Fontan operation.[44] However, conduits used in this setting had several structural, positional, and hemodynamic disadvantages, none of which are shared by the conduits used in the ECF operation. A majority of these conduits were valved homograft or Dacron conduits placed in a retrosternal position, and incorporated the right atrium in the Fontan circuit.[44] The conduits were therefore at significantly higher risk of developing stenosis secondary to the presence of valves in the conduit, use of Dacron for the conduit, compression by the sternum and, importantly, development of turbulence and stasis in the dilated right atrium exposed to elevated systemic venous pressures. In the ECF operation, in contrast, a nonvalved PTFE graft is placed in a posterior location and at little risk for compression. In addition, the ECF conduit maintains laminar flow dynamics by excluding the right atrium, and is therefore at little risk of neointimal peel formation associated with turbulent flow. Marcelletti's group[32] has reported an 18% decrease in luminal diameter of the ECF conduit during the first 6 months after operation, with no subsequent progression during the next 5 years. They have attributed this to use of Dacron instead of PTFE conduits early in their experience. In our experience, none of the patients undergoing an ECF operation has demonstrated evidence of late conduit stenosis or obstruction. We do, nevertheless, recommend periodic imaging to monitor for conduit patency.

THROMBOEMBOLISM

Thromboembolic complications have been reported to occur in as many as 18% to 20% of patients after different types of Fontan procedures.[45,46] In addition, studies have shown that patients with a Fontan circulation have coagulation factor abnormalities that may cause a prothrombotic state.[47,48] Given these findings, and the more extensive use of prosthetic material in the ECF operation, a majority of our patients were discharged from the hospital on acetylsalicylic acid or warfarin. Our current recommendation is warfarin therapy for the first 3 months postoperatively followed by acetylsalicylic acid thereafter. It is important to note, however, that with the ECF approach, in contrast to the lateral tunnel Fontan, prosthetic material and suture lines are avoided entirely from the systemic side of the circulation. This has the important theoretical advantage of decreasing the incidence of left-sided thromboembolism.

SUMMARY

The ECF operation is designed to improve postoperative outcome by enhancing factors that are critical in optimal functioning of the Fontan circulation, including preservation of ventricular and pulmonary vascular function, avoidance of dysrhythmias, and prevention of stasis and flow turbulence in the Fontan circuit. Preoperative strategies include an early bidirectional Glenn procedure, and avoiding ancillary intracardiac procedures at the time of the Fontan by performing them at the time of the Glenn operation. Operative strategies include minimizing the duration of CPB by performing the conduit to pulmonary artery anastomosis off bypass, using partial instead of full CPB by cannulating the IVC alone, avoiding hypothermia, avoiding cross-clamping of the aorta, avoiding atrial incisions and suture lines, using a tubular conduit to construct the Fontan pathway, making a large conduit to pulmonary artery anastomosis, incorporating the conduit into aggressive pulmonary arterioplasties, and offsetting of the superior and inferior cavopulmonary anastomoses.

REFERENCES

1. Fontan F, Kirklin JW, Fernandez G, et al: Outcome after a "perfect" Fontan operation. *Circulation* 81:1520-1536, 1990.
2. Driscoll DJ, Offord KP, Feldt RH, et al: Five- to fifteen-year follow-up after Fontan operation. *Circulation* 85:469-496, 1992.
3. Cetta F, Feldt RH, O'Leary PW, et al: Improved early morbidity and mortality after Fontan operation: The Mayo Clinic experience, 1987 to 1992. *J Am Coll Cardiol* 28:480-486, 1996.
4. Gentles TL, Mayer JE, Gauvreau K, et al: Fontan operation in five hundred consecutive patients: Factors influencing early and late outcome. *J Thorac Cardiovasc Surg* 114:376-391, 1997.
5. Fontan F, Baudet E: Surgical repair of tricuspid atresia. *Thorax* 26:240-246, 1971.
6. de Leval MR, Kilner P, Gewillig M, et al: Total cavopulmonary connection: A logical alternative to atriopulmonary connection for complex Fontan operations. *J Thorac Cardiovasc Surg* 96:682-695, 1988.
7. Puga FJ, Chivarelli M, Hagler DJ: Modification of the Fontan operation applicable to patients with left atrioventricular atresia or single atrioventricular valve. *Circulation* 76:53-60, 1987.
8. Jonas RA, Castaneda AR: Modified Fontan procedure: Atrial baffle and systemic venous to pulmonary artery anastomotic techniques. *J Card Surg* 3:91-96, 1988.
9. Gewillig M, Daenen W, Aubert A, et al: Abolishment of chronic volume overload: Implications for diastolic function of the systemic ventricle immediately after Fontan repair. *Circulation* 86:II-93S-99S, 1992.
10. Caspi J, Coles JG, Rabinowich M, et al: Morphologic findings contributing to a failed Fontan procedure: Twelve-year experience. *Circulation* 82:IV-177S-182S, 1990.
11. Bridges ND, Jones RA, Mayer JE, et al: Bidirectional cavopulmonary anastomosis as interim palliation for high-risk Fontan candidates: Early results. *Circulation* 82:IV-170S-176S, 1990.
12. Jacobs ML, Rychik J, Rome JJ, et al: Early reduction of the volume work of the single ventricle: The hemi-Fontan operation. *Ann Thorac Surg* 62:456-462, 1996.

13. Chang AC, Hanley FL, Wernovsky G, et al: Early bidirectional cavopulmonary shunt in young infants: Postoperative course and early results. *Circulation* 88:149-158, 1993.

14. Reddy VM, McElhinney DB, Moore P, et al: Outcomes after bidirectional cavopulmonary shunt in infants less than 6 months old. *J Am Coll Cardiol* 29:1365-1370, 1997.

15. Billingsley AM, Laks H, Boyce SW, et al: Definitive repair of patients with pulmonary atresia and intact ventricular septum. *J Thorac Cardiovasc Surg* 97:746-754, 1989.

16. Laks H, Pearl JM, Haas GS, et al: Partial Fontan: Advantages of an adjustable interatrial communication. *Ann Thorac Surg* 52:1084-1095, 1991.

17. Bridges ND, Mayer JE, Lock JE, et al: Effect of baffle fenestration on outcome of the modified Fontan operation. *Circulation* 86:1762-1769, 1992.

18. Jacobs ML, Norwood WI: Fontan operation: Influence of modifications on morbidity and mortality. *Ann Thorac Surg* 58:945-952, 1994.

19. Kaulitz R, Ziemer G, Luhmer I, et al: Modified Fontan operation in functionally univentricular hearts: Preoperative risk factors and intermediate results. *J Thorac Cardiovasc Surg* 112:658-664, 1996.

20. Knott-Craig CJ, Danielson GK, Schaff HV, et al: The modified Fontan operation: An analysis of risk factors for early postoperative death or takedown in 702 consecutive patients from one institution. *J Thorac Cardiovasc Surg* 109:1237-1243, 1995.

21. Koutlas TC, Gaynor JW, Nicolson SC, et al: Modified ultrafiltration reduces postoperative morbidity after cavopulmonary connection. *Ann Thorac Surg* 64:37-43, 1997.

22. Balaji S, Gewillig M, Bull C, et al: Arrhythmias after the Fontan procedure: Comparison of total cavopulmonary connection and atriopulmonary connection. *Circulation* 84:III- 162S-167S, 1991.

23. Peters NS, Somerville J: Arrhythmias after the Fontan procedure. *Br Heart J* 68:199-204, 1992.

24. Gelatt M, Hamilton RM, McCrindle BW, et al: Risk factors for atrial tachyarrhythmias after the Fontan operation. *J Am Coll Cardiol* 24:1735-1741, 1994.

25. Gandhi SK, Bromberg BI, Rodefeld MD, et al: Lateral tunnel suture line variation reduces atrial flutter after the modified Fontan operation. *Ann Thorac Surg* 61:1299-1309, 1996.

26. Manning PB, Mayer JE, Wernovsky G, et al: Staged operation to Fontan increases the incidence of sinoatrial node dysfunction. *J Thorac Cardiovasc Surg* 111:833-840, 1996.

27. Fishberger SB, Wernovsky G, Gentles TL, et al: Factors that influence the development of atrial flutter after the Fontan operation. *J Thorac Cardiovasc Surg* 113:80-86, 1997.

28. Humes RA, Feldt RH, Porter CJ, et al: The modified Fontan operation for asplenia and polysplenia syndromes. *J Thorac Cardiovasc Surg* 96:212-218, 1988.

29. Nawa S, Teramoto S: New extension of the Fontan principle: Inferior vena cava–pulmonary artery bridge operation. *Thorax* 43:1022-1023, 1988.
30. Marcelletti C, Corno A, Giannico S, et al: Inferior vena cava-pulmonary artery extracardiac conduit: A new form of right heart bypass. *J Thorac Cardiovasc Surg* 100:228-232, 1990.
31. Giannico S, Corno A, Marino B, et al: Total extracardiac right heart bypass. *Circulation* 86:II-110S-117S, 1992.
32. Amodeo A, Galletti L, Marianeschi S, et al: Extracardiac Fontan operation for complex cardiac anomalies: Seven years' experience. *J Thorac Cardiovasc Surg* 114:1020-1031, 1997.
33. Burke RP, Jacobs JP, Ashraf MH, et al: Extracardiac Fontan operation without cardiopulmonary bypass. *Ann Thorac Surg* 63:1175-1177, 1997.
34. McElhinney DB, Petrossian E, Reddy VM, et al: Extracardiac conduit Fontan procedure without cardiopulmonary bypass. *Ann Thorac Surg* 66:1826-1828, 1998.
35. Van Haesdonck J, Mertens L, Sizaire R, et al: Comparison by computerized numeric modeling of energy losses in different Fontan connections. *Circulation* 92:II-322S-326S, 1995.
36. de Leval MR, Dubini G, Migliavacca F, et al: Use of computational fluid dynamics in the design of surgical procedures: Application to the study of competitive flows in cavopulmonary connections. *J Thorac Cardiovasc Surg* 111:502-513, 1996.
37. Lardo AC, Webber SA, Friehs I, et al: Fluid dynamic comparison of intra-atrial and extracardiac total cavopulmonary connections. *J Thorac Cardiovasc Surg* 117:697-704, 1999.
38. Hsu DT, Quaegebeur JM, Ing FF, et al: Outcome after the single-stage, nonfenestrated Fontan procedure. *Circulation* 96:II-335S-340S, 1997.
39. Laschinger JC, Ringel RE, Brenner JI, et al: Extracardiac total cavopulmonary connection. *Ann Thorac Surg* 54:371-373, 1992.
40. Laschinger JC, Ringel RE, Brenner JI, et al: The extracardiac total cavopulmonary connection for definitive conversion to the Fontan circulation: Summary of early experience and results. *J Card Surg* 8:524-533, 1993.
41. Laschinger JC, Redmond JM, Cameron DE, et al: Intermediate results of the extracardiac Fontan procedure. *Ann Thorac Surg* 68:1261-1267, 1996.
42. Gundry SR, Razzouk AJ, del Rio MJ, et al: The optimal Fontan connection: A growing extracardiac lateral tunnel with pedicled pericardium. *J Thorac Cardiovasc Surg* 114:552-559, 1997.
43. Okabe H, Nagata N, Kaneko Y, et al: Extracardiac cavopulmonary connection of Fontan procedure with autologous pedicled pericardium without cardiopulmonary bypass. *J Thorac Cardiovasc Surg* 116:1073-1075, 1998.
44. Fernandez G, Costa F, Fontan F, et al: Prevalence of reoperation for pathway obstruction after Fontan operation. *Ann Thorac Surg* 48:654-659, 1989.

45. Jahangiri M, Ross DB, Redington AN, et al: Thromboembolism after the Fontan procedure and its modifications. *Ann Thorac Surg* 58:1409-1414, 1994.
46. Rosenthal DN, Friedman AH, Kleinman CS, et al: Thromboembolic complications after Fontan operations. *Circulation* 93:II-287S-293S, 1995.
47. Cromme-Dijkhuis AH, Hess J, Hahlen K, et al: Specific sequelae after Fontan operation at mid- and long-term follow-up. *J Thorac Cardiovasc Surg* 106:1126-1132, 1993.
48. Jahangiri M, Shore D, Kakkar V, et al: Coagulation factor abnormalities after the Fontan procedure and its modifications. *J Thorac Cardiovasc Surg* 113:989-992, 1997.

Index

A

Abciximab, pharmacology, 167

Abiomed Bi-VAD, 112
  illustration showing circulatory
    support with, 113

ACE
  activity in myocardial stunning,
    28
  inhibitors after myocardial
    infarction, 31

Adenosine, and ischemic
    preconditioning, 25

Afterload assessment,
    perioperative imaging for,
    119-120

Agglutinins, cold (*see* Cold
    agglutinins)

Aggrastat, pharmacology, 167

Algorithm, statistical, in surgical
    risk model, 82-84

Allergy to protamine (*see*
    Protamine, allergy to)

Angiotensin-converting enzyme
  activity in myocardial stunning,
    28
  inhibitors after myocardial
    infarction, 31

Anticoagulation, attempted, in
    heparin resistance, 158

Antioxidants, and myocardial
    stunning, 28

Antiplatelet therapy, recent,
    167-168
  perioperative management, 167
  pharmacology, 167

Antithrombin concentrate, in
    management of heparin
    resistance, 159

Antithymocyte preparations, after
    transplantation for
    congenital heart disease,
    69-70

Aortic surgery
  brain injury in
    mechanisms, 2
    monitoring for, 4-5
  cerebral emboli prevention in, 15
  cerebral perfusion in (*see*
    Cerebral, perfusion in aortic
    surgery)
  cerebral protection in (*see*
    Cerebral, protection in aortic
    surgery)

Apoptosis
  in myocardial infarction, 29-30
  in ventricular remodeling, 30-31

Arteriotomy, pulmonary, in right
    ventricular outflow tract
    reconstruction, 170

Artery, coronary artery bypass
    grafting (*see* Coronary, artery
    bypass grafting)

Artifacts, affecting segmental wall
    motion abnormality analysis,
    124

Atrial
  defibrillators (*see* Defibrillators,
    atrial)
  dysrhythmias, reduction with
    extracardiac conduit
    variation of Fontan
    procedure, 185, 189
  flutter, interventional ablative
    therapy for, 108-109
  pacing, dual-site, configuration
    of temporary atrial
    electrodes for, 101